## SURFACE CHANGES

### Normal/smooth

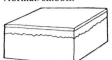

Surface not different from surrounding skin and feels smooth. Stratum corneum and epidermis normal; change in elevation and/or colour only.

### Scaly

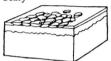

Dry/flaky surface due to abnormal stratum corneum with accumulation of, or increased shedding of, keratinocytes. *Scratch test*: scaly lesions MUST be scratched vigorously with a nail to see if scaling increases and separates easily. If it does the diagnosis is psoriasis.

### Keratin/horn

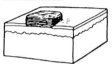

Rough, uneven surface due to accumulation of abnormal keratin. Unlike crust it is difficult to pick off. It is seen on solar keratoses, chronic eczema on the palms and soles, warts and corns.

### Exudate

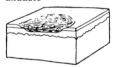

Serum, blood or pus that has accumulated on the surface either from an erosion or ruptured blister/pustule.

### Crust

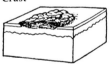

Dried serum, pus or blood. Clinically a crust may be confused with keratin but there should be a history of weeping, pus or bleeding. An attempt should be made to remove the crust to determine whether an ulcer or erosion is underneath.

### Excoriation

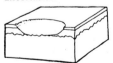

Localized damage to the skin due to scratching. It consists of linear or pinpoint erosions or crusts.

### Warty/papillomatous

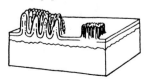

Surface consisting of minute finger-like or round projections.

## TYPES OF LESION

### Macule (size < 1 cm)
### Patch (size > 1 cm)

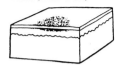

Flat lesions due to local is always normal.

### Papule (size < 1 cm)

Any lesion (< 1 cm) that is raised above the surface or has a scaly, crusted, keratinized or macerated surface.

### Nodule (size > 1 cm)

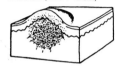

Any elevated lesion (> 1 cm diameter) which has a rounded surface (i.e. the thickness is similar to the diameter): often due to dermal pathology.

### Plaque (size > 1 cm)

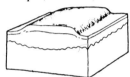

A raised lesion (> 1 cm) where the diameter >> thickness. Usually due to epidermal pathology with scale, crust, keratin or maceration on the surface.

### Vesicle (size < 1 cm)
### Bulla (size > 1 cm)

A fluid-filled lesion (blister).

### Pustule (size < 1 cm)

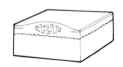

A pus-filled lesion (if in doubt prick lesion and pus comes out). Larger lesions are either abscesses or pseudocysts.

### Erosion

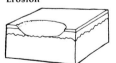

Partial loss of epidermis, which will heal without scarring. Usually secondary to an intraepidermal blister which has burst, and with exudate on the surface.

### Ulcer

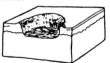

Full thickness loss of epidermis and some dermis, which will heal with scarring. There will be surface exudate (serum, pus or slough) or crust (which should be removed).

# Examples of how to describe clinical features

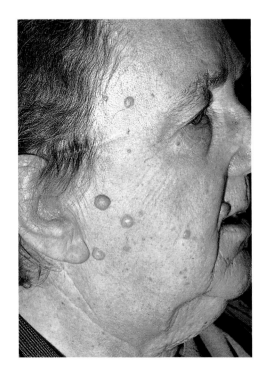

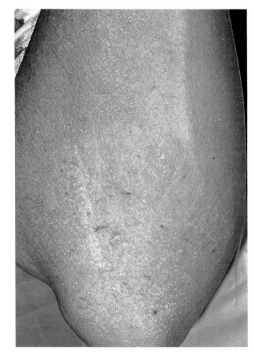

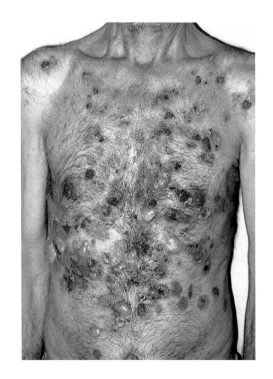

1. Face
2. Non-erythematous
3. Chronic
4. Surface normal/smooth
5. Raised lesions – papules ( < 1 cm)
6. Skin colour

1. Arm (elbow)
2. Erythematous
3. Chronic
4. Surface scaly
5. Raised lesions – plaque ( > 1 cm)
6. Pink colour

1. Trunk
2. Erythematous
3. Chronic
4. Surface exudate/erosions/crusts
5. Raised lesions – bullae and plaques

# Differential Diagnosis in Dermatology

Second Edition

WITH GRATEFUL THANKS TO OUR OWN TEACHERS, KEN, STEPHEN AND JOE

# Differential Diagnosis in Dermatology

Second Edition

**Richard Ashton** *Consultant Dermatologist,*
*Royal Navy Hospital Haslar, Gosport; Honorary Consultant Dermatologist,*
*Royal South Hants Hospital, Southampton, England*

**Barbara Leppard** *Senior Lecturer, Department of Medicine,*
*University of Southampton; Honorary Consultant Dermatologist,*
*Royal South Hants Hospital, Southampton, England*

Foreword by Nicholas J Lowe
*Clinical Professor of Dermatology, UCLA School of Medicine*

RADCLIFFE MEDICAL PRESS · OXFORD

First published 1990
Reprinted 1991
Second edition 1992
Revised reprint 1993

ISBN 1–870905–47–4
ISBN 1–870905–42–3

Library of Congress
Catalog Card Number 89–84267

Printed in Great Britain by
BAS Printers Limited, Over Wallop, Hampshire

# Contents

# Preface to the First Edition

There are many dermatology books on the market, but most of them deal with the subject by diagnosis, with chapters on eczema, psoriasis, etc. This approach is suitable for students and those new to dermatology, but of little use to the doctor when confronted with a patient with an unknown rash. Thus there is a need for a book which provides a guide to dermatological diagnosis in the surgery or clinic. We have tried to provide something that will be of use to the primary care physician, which will sit on his desk and be used day by day.

There are three interlocking components to the book: the algorithms, the descriptive text and the colour photographs; these should be used together in reaching a diagnosis. The chapters are divided into different body areas, and each algorithm deals with the differential diagnosis of similar lesions or rashes, e.g. brown macules or crusted lesions. The possible diagnosis may be confirmed by reading the text describing it and looking at the photographs.

Other diagnostic guides fail to distinguish those conditions which are common from those which are uncommon. It is important to be aware of which diagnoses are the most likely. Within the algorithms, common conditions are printed in white on a strong blue colour, uncommon in black on a lighter shade of blue.

We would like to thank Dr David Jackson for his help with the chapter on the genitalia; the graphics department at Haslar Hospital who prepared the line drawings; the photography department of Haslar Hospital; and Mr White, the medical photographer at the Royal South Hants Hospital, who took many of the clinical photographs.

*January 1990*
Richard Ashton
Barbara Leppard

# Preface to the Second Edition

Despite the proliferation of texts, manuals and atlases on dermatology, it is very gratifying to find that our approach to diagnosis has been so widely accepted. In preparing this revision we have incorporated many of the ideas suggested by reviewers and users of the first edition. As a result, nearly all the algorithms have been changed, some of the illustrations have been replaced and more have been added. Now that it is available in both hardback and limp editions, we hope it will become more accessible to GPs and medical students.

*April 1992*

Richard Ashton
Barbara Leppard

# Foreword

This is an extremely lucid, well-organized and illustrated book that combines excellent clinical photography, practical text and understandable diagrams. Most importantly, the chapters are organized under different skin regions and will assist in the diagnosis of a wide variety of cutaneous diseases. The trainee dermatologist and primary care physician should find it of great value in the evaluation of their dermatologic patients.

The format of this book is such that the reader will be able to follow the necessary steps for the correct identification and diagnosis of the skin disease. They should then be able to decide on either referral for dermatology consultation or choice of therapy by reading an appropriate dermatology text.

The authors are ideally suited for the preparation of this book, having skills and experience in clinical dermatology and teaching. I would like to congratulate them on the high quality of the photographs and illustrations.

*January 1993*

Nicholas J Lowe, MD, FRCP, FACP
*Clinical Professor of Dermatology,*
*UCLA School of Medicine*

# Chapter 1
# Introduction to Dermatological Diagnosis

The diagnosis of skin disease is made by following the same general principles as in any other branch of medicine. Begin by taking a history; this is followed by careful physical examination. If at this stage the diagnosis has not been made, further investigations can be carried out. Very often the non-dermatologist tends to look at a rash or skin lesion and 'guess' the diagnosis. This is quite unnecessary. Below we have outlined a scheme to enable you to make the correct diagnosis most of the time.

## HISTORY TAKING

### PERSONAL HISTORY

#### Time since onset of rash or lesion

This is the most important question in the history. Obviously lesions that have been present for long periods of time need to be distinguished from those that have been present only for a few hours or days.

#### Duration of individual lesions

Do the lesions come or go, and do they occur in the same site or in differing sites? This question is particularly important if the diagnosis of urticaria or herpes simplex is being considered. Urticaria can be diagnosed by the history of lesions coming and going within a 24 hour period. Herpes simplex (and fixed drug eruptions) last around 7−10 days and usually reoccur at the same site.

#### Relationship to physical agents

Ask about relationship to sun exposure in rashes on the face and backs of the hands. Here the important questions are the time after sun exposure before the rash occurs and whether the patient gets the rash on a sunny day through window glass. In solar urticaria the rash occurs within five minutes of sun exposure but is gone in an hour. In polymorphic light eruption the rash occurs several hours after sun exposure and lasts several days. In porphyria (which is very rare) the rash occurs within a few minutes and lasts several days. Rashes that occur through window glass are due to UVA and will not be protected against by ordinary non-opaque sunscreens.

Ask about irritants on the skin in hand eczema, e.g. detergents and oils, and about working practices and hobbies. Are the hands protected by rubber gloves or in direct contact with irritants?

#### Itching or pain

Itching is a helpful symptom but variable. Severe itching, especially at night and preventing sleep, should make you think of scabies (or rarely dermatitis herpetiformis).

#### Size or colour change in pigmented lesions

Get the patient to distinguish between increase in diameter and growing upwards. Superficial malignant melanomas tend to increase in diameter initially, while benign junctional naevi become raised as they turn into compound naevi.

### PAST AND FAMILY HISTORY

#### Past history

Has the patient had a rash before and if so was it the same as now? If eczema is present, a history of infantile eczema, asthma or hay fever may suggest the diagnosis of atopic eczema.

A past history of living or working in a hot climate may be the clue you need for the diagnosis of skin cancer. The following types of skin reaction to sun exposure are recognized:
Type 1: alway burns, never tans;
Type 2: always burns, sometimes tans;
Type 3: sometimes burns, always tans;
Type 4: never burns, always tans.
Those with fair skin (types 1 and 2) are more liable to develop skin cancers with chronic sun exposure.

### Family history

Does anyone else in the family have any skin problem and is it the same as the patient's? This will indicate whether the skin disease is genetically determined, e.g. atopic eczema, ichthyosis or psoriasis; or catching e.g. scabies.

### SOCIAL HISTORY

This should include family relationships and work practices which may give you a clue as to the cause of the problem.

### PREVIOUS TREATMENT

What topical agents have been used e.g. steroids, antibiotics, antifungals or moisturisers, and did they help? It is most important to establish whether these were OINTMENTS or CREAMS, because the base may be as important as the active agent. Remember that local anaesthetics, antibiotics and antihistamines may induce a contact allergic eczema.

A drug history is important if a drug-induced rash is considered.

## DESCRIBING SKIN LESIONS

The following features should be identified in turn:
1 sites involved and distribution;
2 erythematous or non-erythematous;
3 surface characteristics and palpation;
4 types of lesion, including deep palpation;
5 colour;
6 border of rash/lesions and shape;
7 arrangement of lesions;
8 special sites, e.g. scalp, nails, mouth and genitalia.

### 1 SITE AND DISTRIBUTION

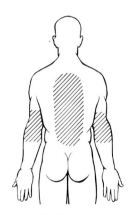 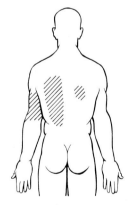

**Symmetrical**

Involving both sides of body to similar extent; usually due to endogeneous causes (e.g. eczema, psoriasis, acne)

**Asymmetrical**

Involving predominantly one side only; usually due to external causes (e.g. bacterial or fungal infections, allergic contact eczema).

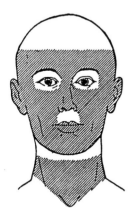 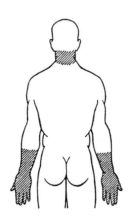

**Sun exposed**

Involving face, 'V' and back of neck, dorsum of hands (forearms). Note behind ears and under chin/eyebrows spared.

## 2 ERYTHEMA

The presence of erythema has been used to distinguish the inflammatory conditions from the others, thus avoiding terms such as rash or lesion, which are difficult to define.

*Erythema* is defined as redness that blanches on pressure, and indicates dilated capillaries. It should be distinguished from *Purpura* which is red, purple, orange or brown, and does not fade on firm pressure; and

*Telangiectasia* which describes small dilated blood vessels visible to the naked eye.

## 3 SURFACE FEATURES

Look and feel the surface. If scaly scratch the surface firmly with

your nail; if crusted remove the crust.

Surface palpation may be divided into:

*smooth*, no irregularity felt;

*uneven*, found with fine scaling or some warty lesions;

*rough*, should feel like sandpaper, and is characteristic of keratin/horn or crust.

**Normal/smooth**

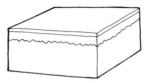

Surface not different from surrounding skin and feels smooth. Stratum corneum and epidermis normal; change in elevation and/or colour only.

**Scaly**

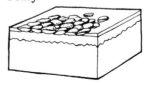

Dry/flaky surface due to abnormal stratum corneum with accumulation of, or increased shedding of, keratinocytes.

*Scratch test*: scaly lesions MUST be scratched vigorously with a nail to see if scaling increases and separates easily. If it does the diagnosis is psoriasis.

**Keratin/horn**

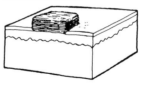

Rough, uneven surface due to accumulation of abnormal keratin. Unlike crust it is difficult to pick off. It is seen on solar keratoses, chronic eczema on the palms and soles, warts and corns.

**Exudate**

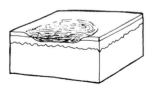

Serum, blood or pus that has accumulated on the surface either from an erosion or ruptured blister/pustule.

**Friable**

Surface bleeds easily after minor trauma.

**Crust**

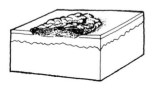

Dried serum, pus or blood. Clinically a crust may be confused with keratin but there should be a history of weeping, pus or bleeding. An attempt should be made to remove the crust to determine whether an ulcer or erosion is underneath.

**Warty/papillomatous**

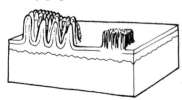

Surface consisting of minute finger-like or round projections.

**Excoriation**

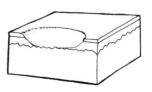

Localized damage to the skin due to scratching and consists of linear or pinpoint erosions or crusts.

**Lichenification**

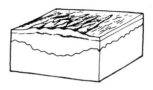

Thickening of the epidermis with increased skin markings due to persistent scratching (found in atopic eczema or lichen simplex).

**Umbilicated**

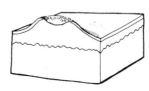

Surface contains a round depression in the centre, characteristic of molluscum contagiosum or herpes simplex.

## 4 TYPES OF LESION

Assess whether the lesions are flat or raised. This may be done by palpation both with finger tips, and deeper palpation using thumb and index finger:

*soft*, feels like the lips;
*normal*, feels like cheeks;
*firm*, feels like tip of nose;
*hard*, feels like forehead.

It is important to assess the depth of the lesion, whether it is sitting on the surface, situated within the dermis or in the subcutaneous tissues. Some lesions may have an *indurated* base, where there is thickening in the depths of the lesion rather than on the surface e.g. a squamous cell carcinoma.

## Primary lesions

**Macule** (size < 1 cm)
**Patch** (size > 1 cm)

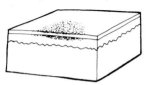

Flat lesions due to localized colour change only; the surface is always normal.

**Papule** (size < 1 cm)

Any lesion (< 1 cm) that is raised above the surface or has a scaly, crusted, keratinized or macerated surface.

**Nodule** (size > 1 cm)

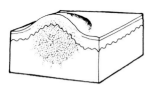

Any elevated lesion (> 1 cm diameter) which has a rounded surface (i.e. the thickness is similar to the diameter): often due to dermal pathology.

**Plaque** (size > 1 cm)

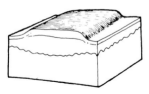

A raised lesion (> 1 cm) where the diameter >> thickness. Usually due to epidermal pathology with scale, crust, keratin or maceration on the surface.

**Vesicle** (size < 1 cm)
**Bulla** (size > 1 cm)

A fluid-filled lesion (blister).

**Pustule** (size < 1 cm)

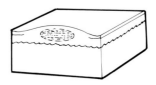

A pus-filled lesion (if in doubt prick lesion and pus comes out). Larger lesions are either abscesses or pseudocysts.

## Secondary lesions

These have developed from primary lesions.

**Erosion**

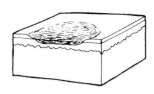

Partial loss of epidermis, which will heal without scarring. Usually secondary to an intraepidermal blister which has burst, and with exudate on the surface.

**Ulcer**

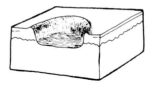

Full thickness loss of epidermis and some dermis, which will heal with scarring. There will be surface exudate (serum, pus or slough) or crust (which should be removed).

## Atrophy

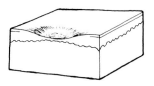

Depression of the surface due to thinning of the epidermis or dermis. Blood vessels are easily seen under the skin, and there is often fine surface wrinkling.

## Fissure

Linear split in epidermis or dermis at an orifice (angle of mouth or anus), over a joint or along a skin crease due to abnormal keratin (usually secondary to eczema). See Fig 8.11, p.214.

## Other terms used

### Weal (=papule/plaque)

Transient swelling due to dermal oedema which should last less than 24 hours at any site — usually synonymous with urticaria.

### Cyst (=papule/nodule)

Cavity lined with epithelium containing fluid, pus or keratin.

### Scar (=macule/papule/plaque)

Healed dermal lesion secondary to trauma, surgery, infection or lack of blood supply.

### Comedone (=papule)

Plugged sebaceous follicle containing altered sebum and cellular debris.

## Burrow (=papule)

Linear 'S' shaped papule 3—5 mm in length found along the sides of fingers or on front of the wrist in patients with scabies.

## 5 COLOUR OF LESION

**Pink/red/purple,** due to blood

Within dilated blood vessels: blanches on pressure=erythema. Outside blood vessels: does not blanche on pressure=purpura. Colour changes from red to purple, to orange brown to brown as haemoglobin is changed to haemosiderin.

**White,** due to loss of pigment

Partial loss of pigment } Distinguished by use of a Wood's
Complete loss of pigment } light (see p. 9).

**Brown,** due to
melanin (see p.12).
haemosiderin following purpura.

**Yellow,** usually due to lipids in the skin.

## 6 BORDER OF LESION OR RASH

**Well defined or circumscribed**

Able to draw a line around the lesion with confidence.

**Poorly defined lesions**

Have border that merges into normal skin or outlying ill-defined papules (characteristic of eczema).

**Active edge**

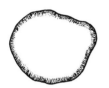

Border of lesion raised or shows increased scaling with relative clearing in centre (characteristic of ringworm).

**Border raised above centre**

Centre of lesion is depressed compared to the edge (characteristic of basal cell carcinoma). See Fig. 5.31, p.146

## SHAPE OF LESION

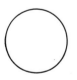

**Round**

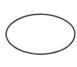

**Oval**

**Irregular**

**Pedunculated**

## 7 ARRANGEMENT OF LESIONS

**Single or multiple**

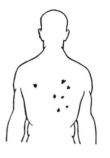

**Discrete**
Separated by normal skin from other similar lesions.

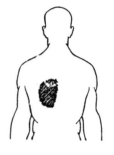

**Unilateral**
Restricted to one side only (herpes zoster, some birthmarks).

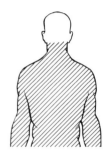

**Generalized**
Covering most of body surface.

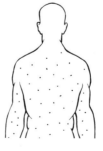

**Disseminated**
Widespread discrete lesions.

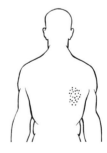

**Grouped**
Multiple lesions grouped in one area.

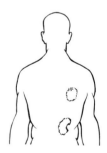

**Annular**
Arranged in a ring.

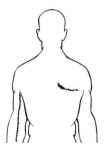

**Linear**

Arranged in line due to:

1   Koebner phenomenon where lesions occur at site of trauma, e.g. linear scratch — psoriasis, lichen planus, warts.
2   Birthmark e.g. epidermal naevus.
3   Confined to a dermatome — herpes zoster.

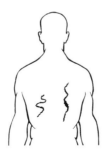

**Serpiginous**

Snake-like.

## SPECIAL INVESTIGATIONS

### WOOD'S LIGHT

This is a source of ultraviolet light from which visible light is excluded by a nickel oxide filter. It is useful in identifying scalp ringworm (p. 23) due to *Microsporum* species which fluoresces green, and erythrasma (p. 182) which fluoresces coral-pink. Porphyrins in urine and faeces fluoresce a bright pink colour. In pigmentary disorders the Wood's light will detect complete loss of pigment in vitiligo (p. 138), incomplete loss in post-inflammatory hypopigmentation and help reveal the extent of pityriasis versicolor (p. 110).

### MYCOLOGY

Fungal infections that you will see on the skin, e.g. dermatophytes (ringworm/tinea), and yeasts such as candida and pityriasis versicolor all live on keratin and can be identified in scales taken from the edge of a scaly lesion. Use a blunt scalpel or banana-shaped blade (Swann major shape 'ʊ', obtainable from Swann-Morton Ltd, Sheffield, S6 2BJ, UK). If the scales are too dry and do not stick to the blade, moistening the skin with surgical spirit helps. The scales can be mixed with 20% KOH (potassium hydroxide) solution to dissolve the keratin, and examined under a microscope; fungal hyphae or yeast spores will be seen (Figs. 1.2 and 1.3)

Alternatively the skin scales may be sent to a mycology laboratory in small opaque envelopes (obtainable from HMSO code no. 27–67), where direct microscopy and culture can be performed (Fig. 1.4).

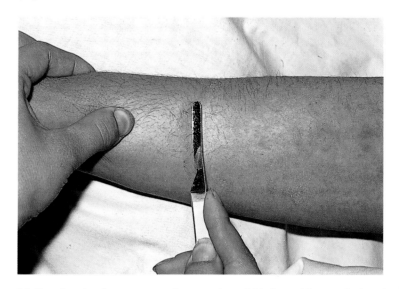

**1.1** Scraping for fungus: use a banana shaped blade or blunt scalpel and scrape from the edge of the lesion.

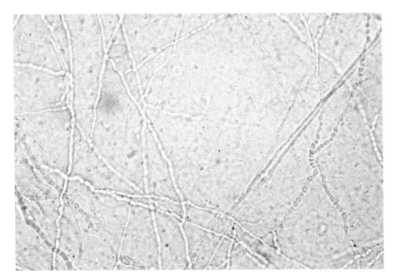

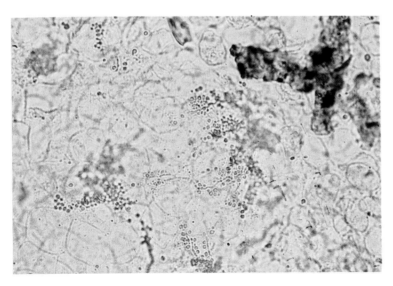

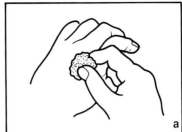

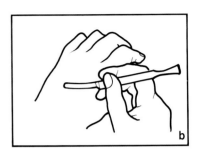

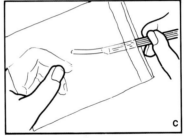

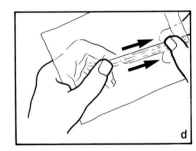

**1.4** How to send samples to the mycology laboratory.

**a** Moisten skin with spirit then allow to dry

**b** To obtain maximum specimen hold scalpel at 15° to skin

**c** Place scalpel blade into self-seal bag

**d** Squeezing blade between fingers, withdraw scalpel

*Left top*
**1.2** Dermatophytes. KOH preparation: direct microscopy showing branching fungal hyphae.

*Left below*
**1.3** Candida. KOH preparation: direct microscopy showing both spores and hyphae. (Courtesy of the Institute of Dermatology).

## PATCH TESTING

This is used to identify a type IV hypersensitivity reaction in the skin, i.e. contact allergic eczema. Possible allergens are applied to the skin of the back on aluminium discs and left in place for 48 hours. A circular plaque of eczema at 48 and 96 hours confined to the area of the disc indicates an allergic response. See Fig. 1.5.

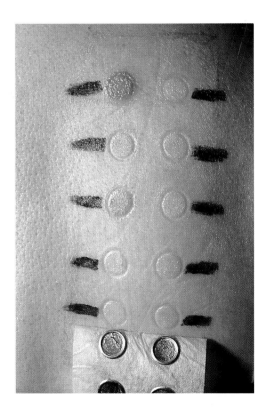

1.5 Patch testing: 48 hour reading. The patches have just been removed and a single test (top left) is positive. Note erythema and vesicles = eczema.

## SKIN BIOPSY

If the diagnosis is in doubt a biopsy can be taken through the edge of the lesion (Fig. 1.6a) so that both normal and abnormal skin are included in the specimen. It should include epidermis, dermis and subcutaneous fat.

If a skin tumour is present, the whole lesion should be excised as an ellipse (Fig. 1.6b) so that the wound can be sewn up in a straight line. Always cut in the direction of the skin lines to get the best cosmetic result.

**1.6** How to perform a skin biopsy.

**a** For diagnosis — elipse through edge of lesion to include normal skin.

**b** Tumour — remove whole lesion with an elipse.

## BACTERIOLOGY AND VIROLOGY CULTURES

Swabs can be taken from vesicles, pustules, erosions or ulcers to identify staphylococci or streptococci by Gram staining of bacteriology culture. Virology cultures are not usually needed, but vesicle fluid can be examined by PAP stain to identify the herpes group of viruses (see Fig. 3.10, p.41), and by electron microscopy if this is available. Virology cultures can also be performed in some laboratories.

# BASIC BIOLOGY OF THE SKIN

The structure of the skin is outlined in Fig. 1.7.

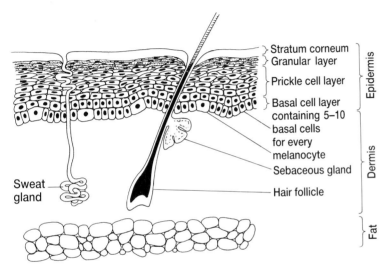

1.7 Structure of the skin.

## THE EPIDERMIS

The epidermis is the outside of the skin. Its function is to produce keratin and melanin. Pathology in the epidermis produces a rash or a lesion with abnormal scale or changes in pigmentation.

### Keratin

Keratin is the end product of maturation of the epidermal cells: its function is to make the skin waterproof.

### Melanin

Melanin is produced by melanocytes in the basal layer. Packets of melanin (melanosomes) are transferred from the melanocytes through their dendritic processes (Fig. 1.8) into the surrounding epidermal cells so that they protect the nucleus from the harmful effects of ultraviolet radiation. Without this protection abnormal cell division occurs leading to skin cancer.

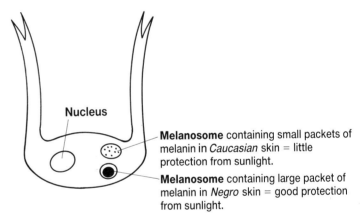

1.8 A melanocyte containing packets of melanin (melanosomes).

## THE DERMIS

The bulk of the dermis is made up of connective tissue; collagen, which gives the skin its strength, and elastic fibres which allow it to stretch. Here are also the blood vessels, lymphatics, cutaneous nerves and the skin appendages (hair follicles, sebaceous glands and sweat glands). Diseases of the dermis usually result in change in elevation of the skin (i.e. papules, nodules, ulcers or atrophy), and if the pathology is restricted to the dermis, there will be no surface changes such as scaling, crust or exudate.

# Chapter 2
# Hairy Scalp

For bald scalp see Chapter 3, p.34

# HAIR PHYSIOLOGY

### WHAT IS HAIR?

Hair is a modified type of keratin produced by the hair matrix (equivalent to epidermis). In man it is largely vestigial since a warm outer covering is not needed. On the scalp, apart from the appearance, its main function is to protect the underlying skin from sun damage.

Three types of hair occur in humans.

1  *Lanugo* hair is the soft silky hair that covers the foetus in utero; it is usually shed before birth.

2  *Vellous* hair is the short fine hair which covers the whole skin surface apart from palms and soles.

3  *Terminal* hair is longer, coarser, and pigmented. Before puberty terminal hair is restricted to the scalp, eyebrows and eyelashes; after puberty secondary terminal hair develops in response to androgens in the axillae, pubic area and on the front of the chest in men.

### HAIR CYCLE

There are between 100,000 and 150,000 hairs on the scalp. The hair cycle (Fig. 2.1) occurs randomly in each follicle over the scalp so that up to 100 hairs are being lost daily, but in normal circumstances moulting does not occur.

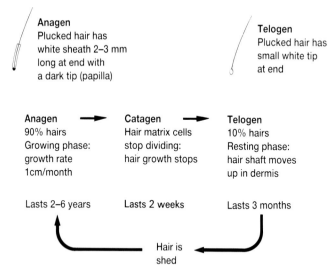

2.1 Hair cycle.

# HAIR LOSS

If the patient is complaining of hair loss, *first find out exactly what they mean*:

1  Patient has noticed increased number of hairs falling out each day over a short period of time (1–2 months), but there are no bald areas: see p. 15.

2  Patient seems to have less hair than before and may or may not have noticed hair coming out over a period of months or years: see p. 16.

3  Hair has become finer: see p. 16.

4  Discrete bald areas are visible. Look to see if the scalp is normal, scaly or scarred. If there is no scarring see p. 19.
If scarring is present see p. 24.

5  All the scalp hair and/or body hair has disappeared: see p. 19.

6  Hair breaks easily and will not grow to the desired length: see p.26.

## ANAGEN EFFLUVIUM

Cytotoxic drugs affect any rapidly dividing cells and the hair matrix is affected as well as the bone marrow and tumour cells. It is the anagen hairs that are shed so 90 percent of all scalp hair will be lost.

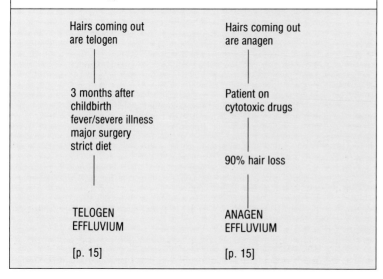

**Diffuse hair loss**
**1 Patient has noticed increased number of hairs falling out each day over a short period of time (1−2 months), but there are no bald areas**

| Hairs coming out are telogen | Hairs coming out are anagen |
|---|---|
| 3 months after childbirth fever/severe illness major surgery strict diet | Patient on cytotoxic drugs |
| | 90% hair loss |
| TELOGEN EFFLUVIUM | ANAGEN EFFLUVIUM |
| [p. 15] | [p. 15] |

## TELOGEN EFFLUVIUM

During pregnancy the hair cycle stops. At the time of delivery all the hairs that should have gone into telogen during the previous 9 months do so. Three months later these telogen hairs are shed and considerable hair loss occurs. The hair will often come out in handfuls when you pull gently on the hair. Since shedding of telogen hairs is followed by regrowth of anagen hair, such hair loss is short lived and fully reversible. Similar shedding of telogen hairs can occur three months after any severe illness, major operation or very strict dieting.

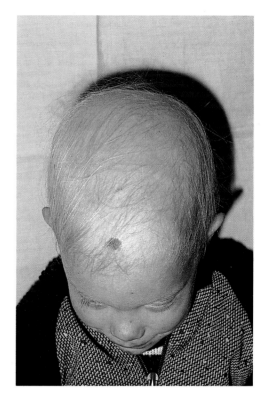

**2.2** Anagen effluvium in a 3 year old boy having chemotherapy.

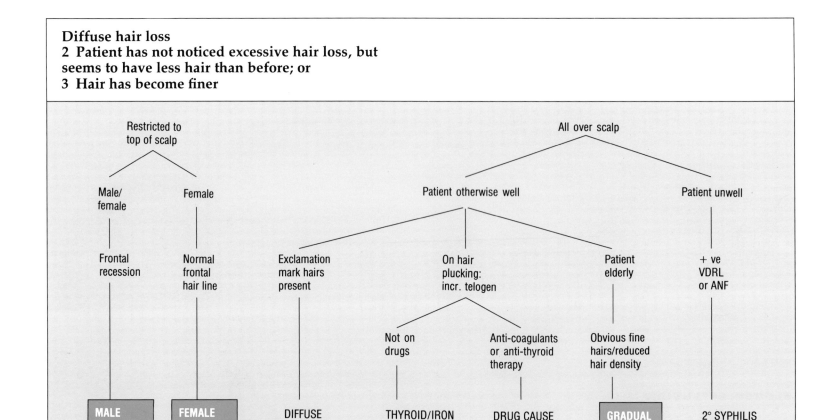

**Diffuse hair loss**
**2 Patient has not noticed excessive hair loss, but seems to have less hair than before; or**
**3 Hair has become finer**

Restricted to top of scalp → Male/female → Frontal recession → **MALE PATTERN ALOPECIA** [p. 16]

Restricted to top of scalp → Female → Normal frontal hair line → **FEMALE PATTERN ALOPECIA** [p. 17]

All over scalp → Patient otherwise well → Exclamation mark hairs present → DIFFUSE ALOPECIA AREATA [p. 18]

All over scalp → Patient otherwise well → On hair plucking: incr. telogen → Not on drugs → THYROID/IRON DEFICIENCY [p. 18]

All over scalp → Patient otherwise well → On hair plucking: incr. telogen → Anti-coagulants or anti-thyroid therapy → DRUG CAUSE [p. 18]

All over scalp → Patient otherwise well → Patient elderly → Obvious fine hairs/reduced hair density → **GRADUAL HAIR LOSS WITH AGE** [p. 18]

All over scalp → Patient unwell → + ve VDRL or ANF → 2° SYPHILIS or S.L.E. [p. 18]

## MALE PATTERN BALDNESS

This is hair loss occurring over the temples or on the crown: the hair on the occiput and around the sides of the scalp is never lost. It can only occur when androgens are present, but it does not mean there is an excess in either male or female patients. An

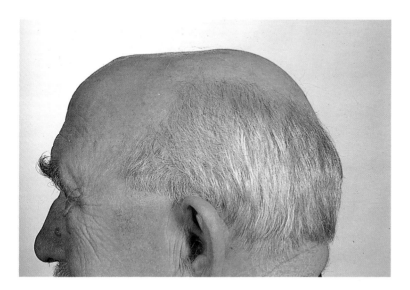

**2.3** Male pattern alopecia.

## OTHER CAUSES OF DIFFUSE HAIR LOSS

### When the hair density looks normal

Many patients complain that they have less hair than they would like, but there is no abnormality to be found on clinical examination. Plucking a group of hairs with a pair of artery forceps and counting the proportion of growing/resting (anagen/telogen) hairs will tell you whether to investigate the patient further. If the

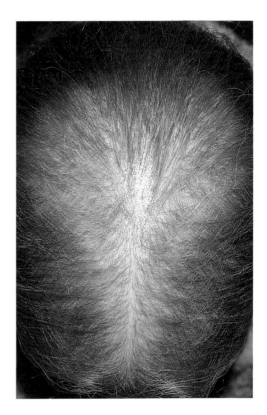

**2.4** Female pattern baldness.

androgen-secreting tumour should be considered in a woman if the alopecia is very extensive or if there is a change in the menstrual cycle.

The first change that occurs is a shift in the hair cycle towards telogen, i.e. there is an increase in telogen hairs. Gradually the hair follicles get smaller and terminal hairs are replaced by vellous hairs. The amount of hair loss and the age of onset in men is genetically determined.

## FEMALE PATTERN BALDNESS

This is similar to the male pattern but without the frontal recession. Decreased hair density from the crown forward with normal hair density at the back and sides occurs. Minor degrees of this are extremely common.

percentage of telogen hairs is increased to 30–50, instead of 10, check that the patient is not hypothyroid, iron deficient or taking anti-coagulant or anti-thyroid drugs.

**When the hair density is obviously reduced (Fig. 2.5)**

The hair density gradually decreases with age and the hairs become finer. In younger patients consider hypothyroidism, iron deficiency, and diffuse alopecia areata (look for ! hairs). If the patient is unwell consider secondary syphilis or systemic lupus erythematosus.

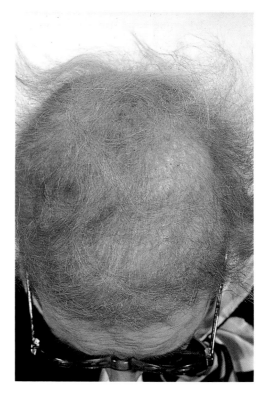

**2.5** Diffuse hair loss in a 60 year old lady.

## 4a Discrete bald areas — without scarring
## 5 Complete hair loss

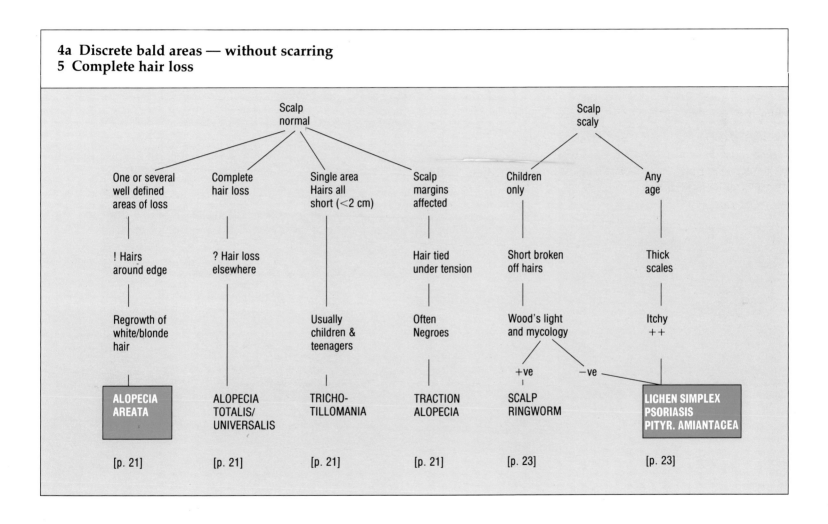

Scalp normal

| | | | |
|---|---|---|---|
| One or several well defined areas of loss | Complete hair loss | Single area Hairs all short (<2 cm) | Scalp margins affected |
| ! Hairs around edge | ? Hair loss elsewhere | | Hair tied under tension |
| Regrowth of white/blonde hair | | Usually children & teenagers | Often Negroes |
| **ALOPECIA AREATA** | ALOPECIA TOTALIS/ UNIVERSALIS | TRICHO-TILLOMANIA | TRACTION ALOPECIA |
| [p. 21] | [p. 21] | [p. 21] | [p. 21] |

Scalp scaly

| | |
|---|---|
| Children only | Any age |
| Short broken off hairs | Thick scales |
| Wood's light and mycology | Itchy ++ |
| +ve / −ve | |
| SCALP RINGWORM | **LICHEN SIMPLEX PSORIASIS PITYR. AMIANTACEA** |
| [p. 23] | [p. 23] |

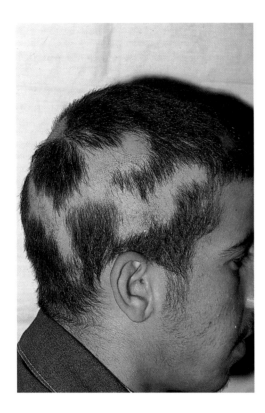

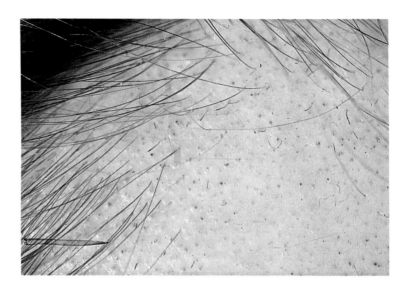

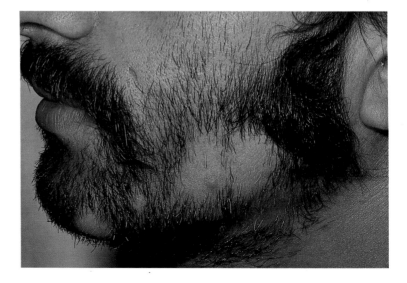

*Left*
**2.6** Alopecia areata: discrete bald patches, but no erythema or scaling.

*Right above*
**2.7** Alopecia areata: exclamation mark hairs at edge of bald patch.

*Right below*
**2.8** Alopecia areata of beard area.

## ALOPECIA AREATA

This is the commonest cause of discrete hair loss in both children and adults. There is no redness or scaling of the underlying scalp. It lasts usually for 3–6 months and then the hair regrows spontaneously. While the disease is active ! hairs will be seen around the edge of the bald patches: these are short broken-off hairs where the broken end is thicker and darker than where the hair emerges from the scalp. Only pigmented hairs are affected, so normal white/grey hairs can be seen in the middle of a bald area. When the hair regrows it is white for the first 6–8 weeks. There may be one or several bald patches on the scalp or any other hairy area.

Alopecia areata is renamed *alopecia totalis* when all hair is lost from the scalp and *alopecia universalis* if both scalp and body hair are absent.

## TRACTION ALOPECIA

This is uncommon: it is due to the hair being tightly pulled back and tied up, or too tightly rolled or straightened with hot combs.

## TRICHOTILLOMANIA

This is a well-defined area of apparent hair loss. Close examination will reveal not a bald area, but an area where all the hairs are short, longer hair having been pulled out. The remaining hair is just too short to twist around the fingers to pull out. It usually occurs in children or teenagers who are unhappy, and gets better when things improve.

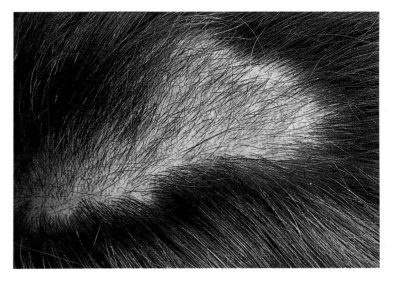

**2.9** Trichotillomania: looks like a bald patch but in fact short hairs are present.

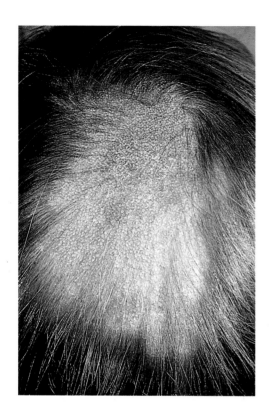

**2.10** Tinea capitis (scalp ringworm): discrete bald patch with scaly surface.

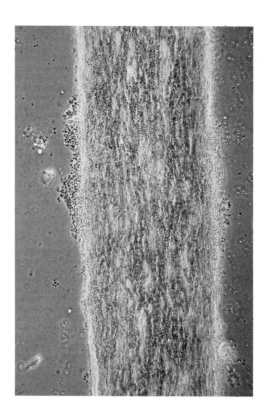

**2.11** Tinea capitis: direct microscopy of affected hair showing small spores both inside hair shaft and outside — typical of microsporum infection.

## SCALP RINGWORM

Scalp ringworm only occurs in children: it is not a cause of hair loss in adults. It is due to one of two organisms, *Microsporum canis* (caught from kittens or puppies) and *Microsporum audouinii* (caught from other children). Discrete bald areas in which the underlying skin is red and scaly, together with a history of other children with similar hair loss or a new kitten or puppy whose fur is falling out make the diagnosis likely. It can be proved by seeing green fluorescence under a Wood's light (ultra-violet light), identifying the spores on direct microscopy of the hair, or by culturing the organism from plucked hairs. On rare occasions the animal variety may produce a red boggy mass (kerion).

## SKIN DISEASE AFFECTING THE SCALP

Eczema and psoriasis should not cause hair loss, but if very itchy, the hairs may be broken off by continual rubbing and scratching. Both conditions may rarely cause thick scales which grow out along the hairs (pityriasis amiantacea) and the hairs may be broken off with the scale.

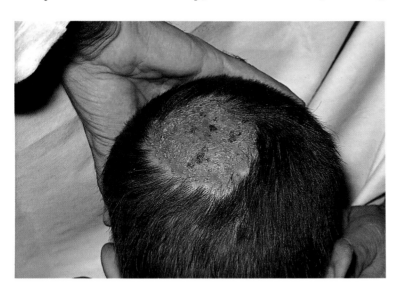

**2.12** Tinea capitis: kerion — a boggy inflammatory swelling due to animal ringworm.

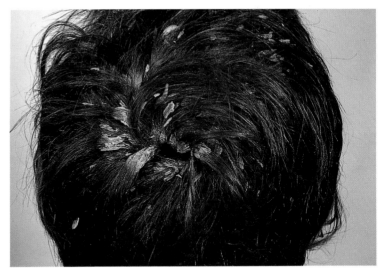

**2.13** Pityriasis amiantacea. This may be due to eczema or psoriasis. The scales grow out along the hairs.

## 4b  Discrete bald areas — with scarring
**All these causes are uncommon. The hair follicles are replaced by scar tissue or tumour, so hair loss is permanent.**

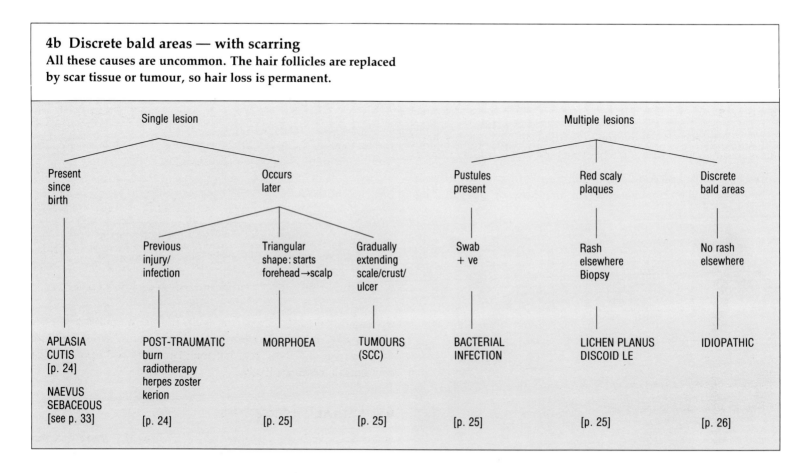

### APLASIA CUTIS

Presents at birth as an ulcerated red area: this heals to leave permanent scarring (see also naevus sebaceous p. 33).

### POST TRAUMATIC

Any injury or infection resulting in scarring will result in hair loss. Ringworm in this country does not cause scarring, but in some parts of the world where Favus occurs (e.g. Middle East) permanent alopecia may develop.

## MORPHOEA

Linear morphoea affecting the frontal area may also involve the scalp, with subsequent hair loss (see p. 149).

## TUMOURS

Scalp hair protects the skin from sun damage, so tumours here mainly occur in men who have become bald at an early age. Basal

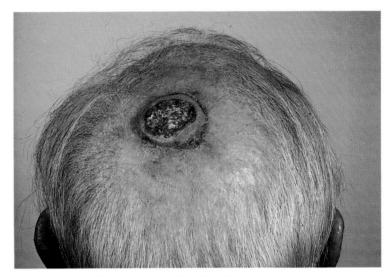

**2.15** Squamous cell carcinoma on the bald scalp in a man in his seventies.

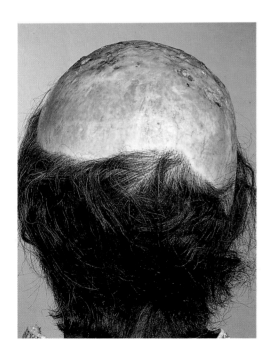

**2.14** Traumatic alopecia following a burn in childhood.

cell carcinomas are rare on the scalp unless the patient has previously had radiotherapy (for treating ringworm before the introduction of griseofulvin in 1958): solar keratoses and squamous cell carcinomas are more likely.

## BACTERIAL INFECTIONS

Folliculitis decalvans is a rare condition in which there is a slow spread of scarring folliculitis across the scalp due to infection with *Staphylococcus aureus*.

## LICHEN PLANUS AND DISCOID LUPUS ERYTHEMATOSUS

The diagnosis of these can usually be made from the rash elsewhere

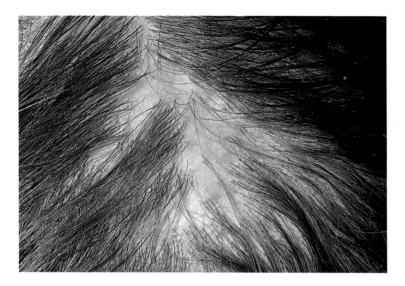

**2.16** Scarring alopecia on the scalp due to lichen planus.

(see pp. 68 and 94). If the scalp alone is affected a biopsy is needed.

## IDIOPATHIC

In many patients there is no obvious cause for the hair loss.

# 6 Structural Abnormalities of Hair

The patient has noticed that hair breaks easily and will not grow to the desired length. There are numerous structural abnormalities of the hair shaft which cause hair to break off short. All are extremely rare.

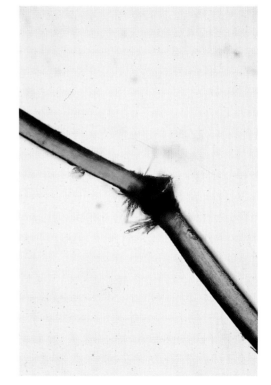

**2.17** Trichorrhexis nodosa: small nodular swellings occur along the hair shaft and the hair breaks at these points.
This is just one example of the numerous structural abnormalities that stop the hair growing long.

# EXCESSIVE HAIR

Hair in the wrong place or hair which is coarser or longer than socially acceptable is regarded as excessive. There are two different patterns:

1 *Hirsutism*. In women, coarse terminal hair in the moustache or beard area, and on the chest or lower abdomen as in men, is known as hirsutism. It is extremely common, the amount of hair being genetically determined.

2 *Hypertrichosis* is excessive hair all over the body. Either the foetal lanugo hair is not lost before birth or regrows at some later stage. When confined to the lumbosacral area it may be a marker of an underlying spina bifida.

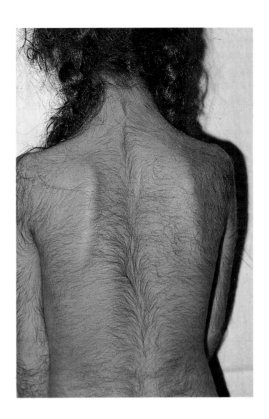

**2.19** Hypertrichosis.

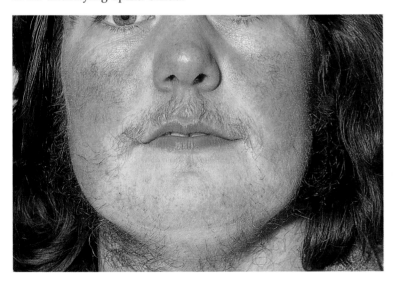

**2.18** Hirsutism.

## RASHES AND LESIONS IN THE HAIRY SCALP

**Hairy scalp**
**Itch/scaling with/without erythema/crusting**

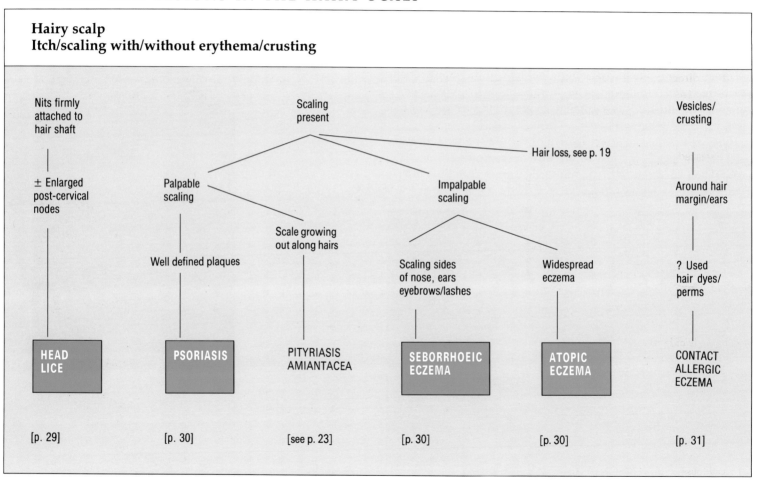

Nits firmly attached to hair shaft

Scaling present

Hair loss, see p. 19

Vesicles/crusting

± Enlarged post-cervical nodes

Palpable scaling

Impalpable scaling

Around hair margin/ears

Well defined plaques

Scale growing out along hairs

Scaling sides of nose, ears eyebrows/lashes

Widespread eczema

? Used hair dyes/perms

**HEAD LICE**

**PSORIASIS**

PITYRIASIS AMIANTACEA

**SEBORRHOEIC ECZEMA**

**ATOPIC ECZEMA**

CONTACT ALLERGIC ECZEMA

[p. 29]   [p. 30]   [see p. 23]   [p. 30]   [p. 30]   [p. 31]

## HEAD LICE (PEDICULOSIS CAPITIS)

Lice are wingless insects which pierce the skin to feed on human blood. The head louse is about 3 mm long and the female lays 7–10 eggs each day during a life span of one month (Fig. 2.20). Spread by direct contact from head to head, mainly in children, it has nothing to do with poor hygiene. The eggs are firmly attached to the base of the hair, and hatch in about a week. Infestation is extremely common and usually asymptomatic, but if there are large numbers of lice, itching may be intolerable and result in secondary bacterial infection (impetigo and pustules). Enlarged posterior cervical glands should always make you think of head lice. The diagnosis is made by finding the nits (egg cases), which are white opalescent oval capsules, firmly attached to hairs (unlike dandruff where the scale easily comes off).

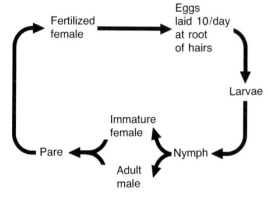

2.20 Life cycle of head louse

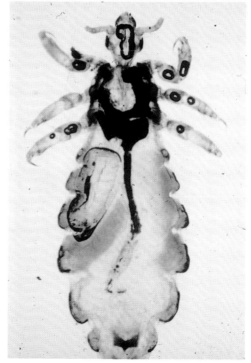

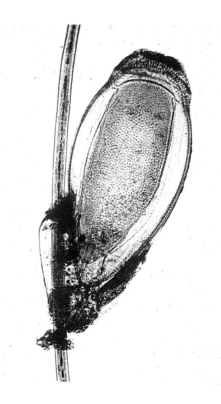

*Right*
**2.21** Head louse: fertilised female (× 50).

*Far right*
**2.22** Head louse nit (egg) firmly cemented onto hair shaft (× 40).

## PSORIASIS

Psoriasis in the scalp is common, and it may first begin there. The diagnosis is made by running your hands through the scalp and feeling the thick heaped up scales, which accumulate because of the hair. On examination the lesions are identical to those found elsewhere i.e. discrete, red scaly plaques.

## ECZEMA

Eczema is differentiated from psoriasis on the scalp because it usually covers all the hairy scalp and is more easily seen than felt: wherever you look it is red and scaly. Any type of eczema can affect the scalp, but particularly atopic and seborrhoeic (see pp. 103 and 106).

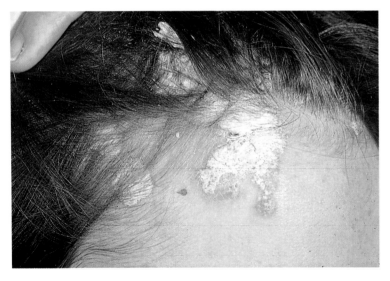

**2.23** Psoriasis: thick heaped up scale in hairy scalp spreading onto forehead.

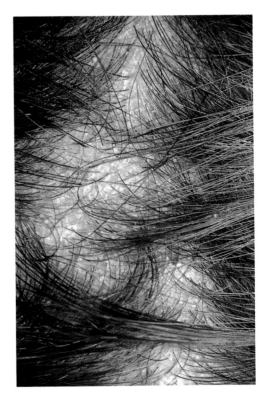

**2.24** Seborrhoeic eczema: fine scaling all over scalp. Ordinary dandruff is mild seborrhoeic eczema.

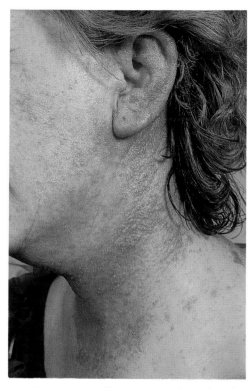

**2.25** Acute contact allergic eczema due to hair dye affecting the ears. A similar picture could be due to antibiotic or antihistamine ear drops.

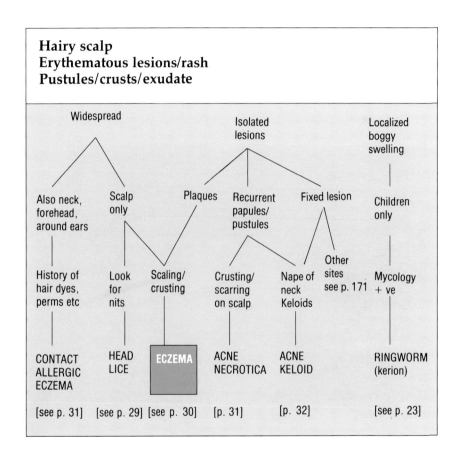

confirmed once the patient is better by patch testing.

## CONTACT ALLERGIC ECZEMA

Contact allergic eczema on the scalp is not common and is usually due to hair dyes (paraphenylene diamine), or perming solutions (thioglycollates). It presents as an acute weeping eczema at the hair margins and on the forehead, face and neck. The diagnosis is

## ACNE NECROTICA

It is not related to acne. This condition occurs in adult men and presents as itchy or painful papules and pustules, which crust over and heal leaving scars. The cause is unknown.

## ACNE KELOID

This is a chronic inflammatory condition on the nape of the neck, most commonly seen in Negro men. Itchy follicular pustules develop in the occipital area which heal to leave keloid scars; the cause is unknown.

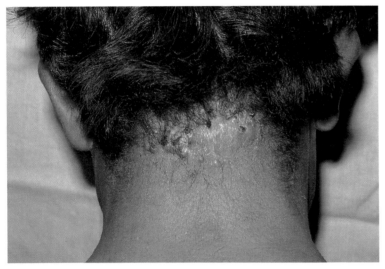

**2.26** Acne Keloid.

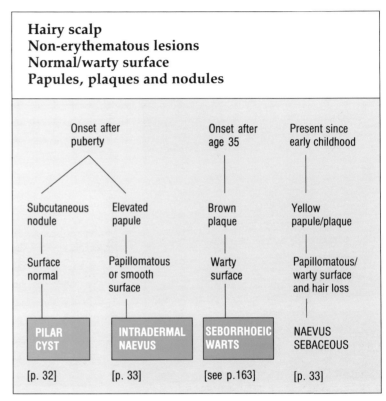

## PILAR CYSTS

Pilar (or trichilemmal) cysts are derived from the external root sheath of hair follicles and occur predominantly on the scalp. They are inherited as an autosomal dominant trait, appear between the ages of 15 and 30, and present to the doctor because the patient notices a lump when brushing or combing the hair. One or several subcutaneous nodules are present. They do not have a

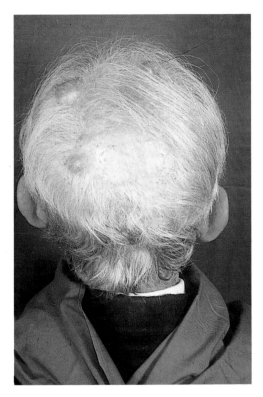

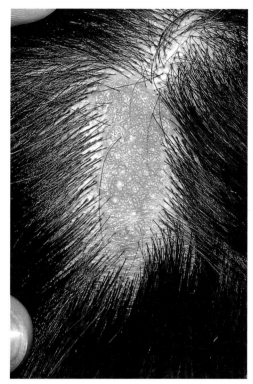

*Right*
**2.27** Multiple pilar cysts on scalp.

*Far right*
**2.28** Naevus sebaceous: present since birth.

punctum and do not usually become inflamed (compare with epidermoid cysts. p. 150).

## NAEVUS SEBACEOUS

These are present from early childhood. They differ from moles in being yellowish with a warty surface and having hair loss over them. If left they may sometimes develop basal cell carcinomas within them in middle age.

## INTRADERMAL NAEVUS

Flat pigmented naevi are not usually recognized on the scalp. Once they become raised they are likely to be caught in combs. Most skin coloured or slightly brown papules in the scalp will be intradermal naevi. They may have a smooth or papillomatous surface (see p. 147).

# Chapter 3
# Erythematous Rashes and Lesions on the Face

## ACUTE

**Face**
**Acute erythematous rash/lesions**
**Normal/smooth surface**
**Widespread patches/papules/plaques/swelling**

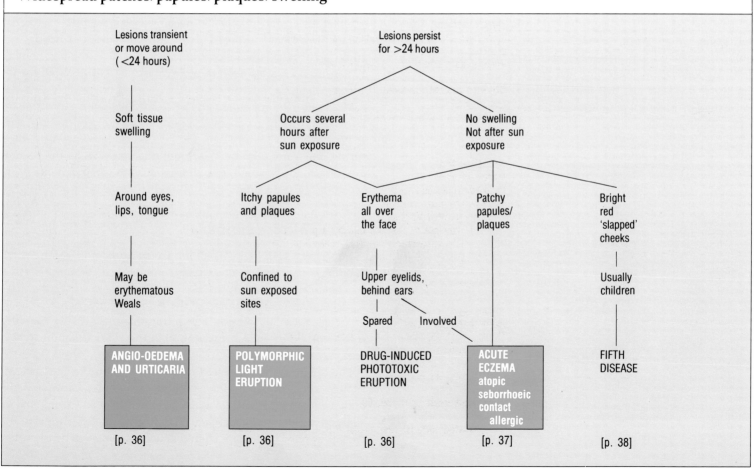

| | | | | |
|---|---|---|---|---|
| Lesions transient or move around (<24 hours) | | Lesions persist for >24 hours | | |

Soft tissue swelling — Occurs several hours after sun exposure / No swelling Not after sun exposure

- Around eyes, lips, tongue
- Itchy papules and plaques
- Erythema all over the face
- Patchy papules/ plaques
- Bright red 'slapped' cheeks

- May be erythematous Weals
- Confined to sun exposed sites
- Upper eyelids, behind ears (Spared / Involved)
- Usually children

**ANGIO-OEDEMA AND URTICARIA** [p. 36]

**POLYMORPHIC LIGHT ERUPTION** [p. 36]

DRUG-INDUCED PHOTOTOXIC ERUPTION [p. 36]

**ACUTE ECZEMA** atopic seborrhoeic contact allergic [p. 37]

FIFTH DISEASE [p. 38]

## ANGIO-OEDEMA

Angio-oedema is due to swelling of the dermis resulting from increased permeability of blood vessels (see urticaria p. 72). On the face the swelling involves the eyelids and lips. Less commonly the tongue and larynx may be involved leading to difficulty in swallowing and breathing. The onset is dramatic and may make the patient feel ill with closure of the eyes. The swelling should start going down quite quickly, but can last up to 48 hours. If there is associated urticaria the diagnosis is easy. When it occurs alone it needs to be distinguished from contact allergic eczema and erysipelas. The fact that the swelling is not red and there are no blisters or scaling should make diagnosis easy.

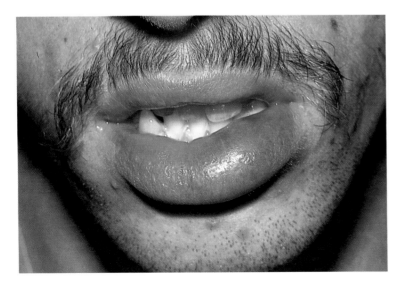

**3.1** Angio-oedema of the lower lip.

## POLYMORPHIC LIGHT ERUPTION

This is a common rash due to ultraviolet light. It occurs in early adult life and affects twice as many females as males. The eruption consists of itchy red papules, vesicles or plaques. The size of the papules varies in different patients from pin point up to 5 mm. The plaques may be urticarial (i.e. non-scaly dermal oedema) or eczematous (scaly, poorly defined). Vesicles are less common. It occurs only on sun exposed parts, especially back of hands, forearms, 'V' of neck and below the ears, as well as the face, but not all sun-exposed sites need to be involved, and quite often the face may be clear.

Most patients are aware of the connection with sun exposure. The rash typically occurs after a delay of several hours and if there is no further exposure lasts for 2–5 days. It occurs initially in spring and early summer, and tends to improve as the summer progresses due to some form of tolerance. In some patients it only occurs away from home (on holiday) in more intense sunlight.

## PHOTOTOXIC RASHES

A phototoxic rash looks like sunburn but occurs in a patient who has not been exposed to excessive sunlight. It is caused by:
1   chemicals applied to the skin, e.g. psoralens in suncreams;
2   accidental contamination of the skin by wood tars in creosote;
3   drugs taken by mouth, e.g. tetracylines (especially dimethyl-chlortetracyline), chlorpromazine, chlorthiazides, thiazide diuretics and psoralens.

The diagnosis is suggested by the distribution of the rash with shaded sites (upper eyelids, behind ears, under chin) spared. It may be confused with contact allergic eczema to an airborne allergen or an applied cream. The history of drug ingestion or creams applied to the face should enable the cause to be identified.

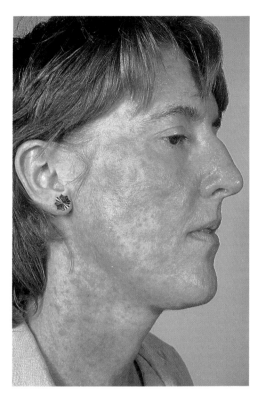

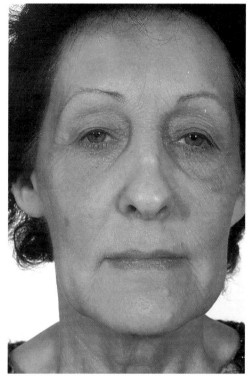

*Right*
**3.2** Polymorphic light eruption: itchy papules and vesicles on the face.

*Far right*
**3.3** Acute eczema due to lanolin sensitivity. No obvious vesicles or scaling; the rash merges imperceptibly into the normal skin.

## ACUTE ECZEMA

Acute eczema may occur without obvious vesicles. It consists of itchy erythematous small pinhead papules that coalesce to form plaques. After several days mild scaling should be evident. The most notable characteristic of eczema is that the border of the rash is ill defined merging imperceptibly into normal skin. The surface often shows minute erosions and crusts where microvesicles have burst and crusted over. These features will suggest a diagnosis of acute eczema, and the ill-defined distribution will tend to exclude the other conditions mentioned above.

On the face, acute eczema may be the result of a flare up of chronic atopic or seborrhoeic eczema, or be a contact allergic eczema (see pp. 45, 103 and 106).

**3.4** Acute eczema. Pinhead papules and crusts on the upper back of a patient with a contact allergic eczema to a topical antihistamine.

## FIFTH DISEASE (ERYTHEMA INFECTIOSUM/ SLAPPED CHEEK DISEASE)

This viral disease is characterized by the appearance of red papules on the cheeks which coalesce within hours to form symmetrical, red, oedematous plaques sparing the nasolabial folds and eyelids. Symptoms are mild (sore throat, pruritis, fever) or absent. The 'slapped cheek appearance' fades in 4 days, but within 48 hours of the onset of the facial erythema, a lace-like pattern of erythema appears on the proximal limbs extending to trunk and extremities. This fades within 6–14 days.

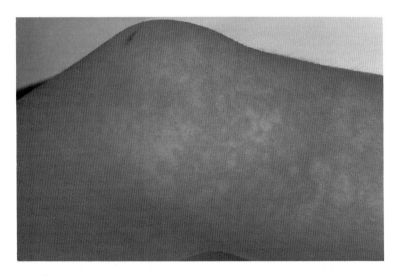

**3.5** Fifth disease: lace-like pattern on the leg.

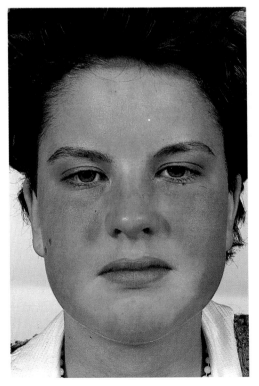

**3.6** Fifth disease: typical 'slapped cheek appearance'.

**Face, trunk, limbs**
**Acute erythematous rash/lesions**
**Blisters/exudate/crusts/erosions**
**1 Localized**

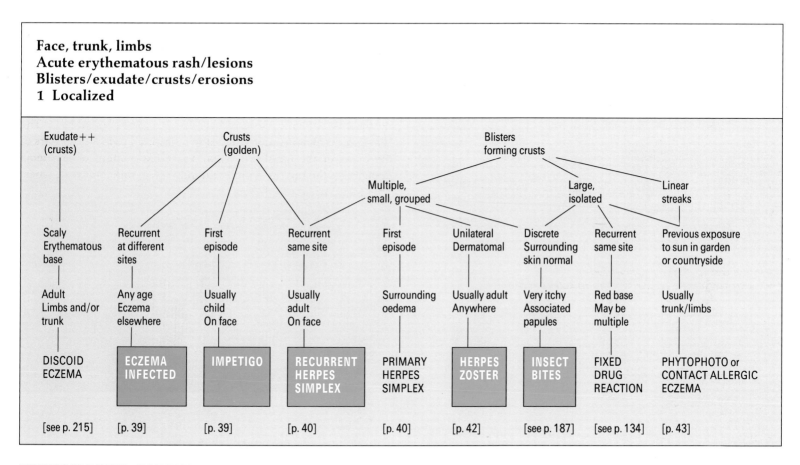

## IMPETIGINIZED ECZEMA

Any form of eczema may become secondarily infected with *Staphylococcus aureus* once the skin has been broken by scratching. Weeping occurs and a golden yellow crust appears on the surface. The diagnosis is made by the preceding history of eczema, although an isolated plaque may be difficult to differentiate from impetigo.

## IMPETIGO

This is a very superficial infection of the epidermis with *Staphylococcus aureus*, a group A beta-haemolytic streptococcus or a mixture of both. Mainly children are infected since the organisms gain entry through broken skin (cuts and grazes): it is very contagious. Typically it starts as small vesicles which rapidly break

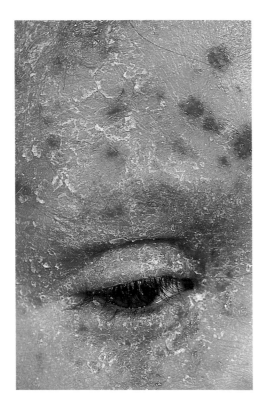

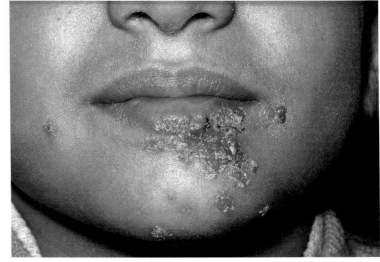

**3.7** Impetiginized atopic eczema in a 4-year-old girl.

**3.8** Impetigo: typical honey-coloured crusts.

down to form golden yellow crusts; less commonly there may be just a glazed erythema.

## PRIMARY HERPES SIMPLEX

Infection with the *Herpes hominis* virus type 1 most commonly affects the buccal mucosa and occurs in the first five years of life. It is usually asymptomatic but may cause an acute gingivo-stomatitis, or painful blistering on any part of the skin (grouped blisters occurring on an oedematous background. The diagnosis may be confirmed by a PAP stain of the contents of a blister when multinucleate giant cells are seen (Fig. 3.10).

## RECURRENT HERPES SIMPLEX

Recurrent herpes simplex usually affects the lips if the primary infection was in the mouth, or the same site as the primary infection if that was on the skin surface. It is preceded by a

**3.9** Primary herpes simplex infection on the right cheek. Grouped vesicles which have burst to form crusts associated with marked surrounding oedema.

*Far right above*
**3.10** PAP stain of vesicle fluid from primary or secondary herpes simplex. Multinucleate giant cells are indicative of any herpes infection (simplex or zoster).

*Far right, below*
**3.11** Recurrent herpes simplex on and below the lower lip.

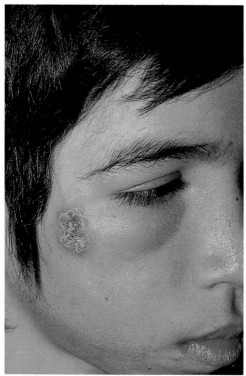

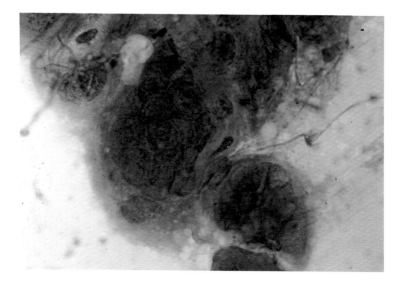

prodromal sensation of itching, burning or tingling. Small grouped vesicles appear, burst, crust and then heal in 7–10 days without scarring. The vesicles are due to disruption of epidermal cells by viral multiplication within them. Factors precipitating recurrent episodes are fever (hence the name 'cold sores'), sunlight, menstruation and stress. These episodes can continue throughout life.

Herpes simplex may be differentiated from impetigo by the history of recurrent episodes, prodromal pain and initial vesicles containing clear fluid, and in adults is the more likely diagnosis.

## HERPES ZOSTER

Herpes zoster occurs in people who have previously had chicken pox. The virus, *Herpes varicella-zoster*, lies dormant in the dorsal root ganglion following chicken pox, and later travels down the cutaneous nerves to infect the epidermal cells. Destruction of these cells results in the formation of intra-epidermal vesicles.

For several days before the rash appears, there is pain or an abnormal sensation in the skin. Then comes the rash: groups of

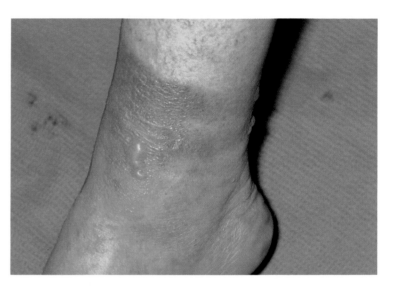

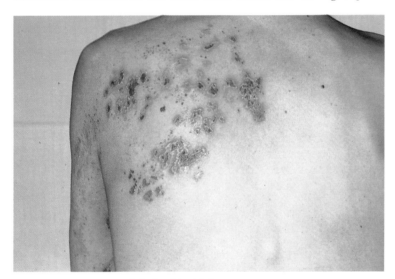

**3.12** Herpes zoster over left shoulder blade.

*Right above*
**3.13** Phytophotodermatitis on the ankle and foot of a patient who has been using a strimmer whilst wearing long trousers and sandals.

*Right below*
**3.14** Contact allergic eczema on the forearm due to *Primula obconica*; note the linear blisters.

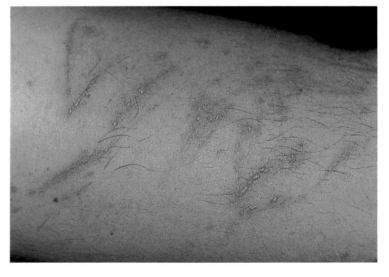

small vesicles on a red background. Weeping and crusting then occur and healing takes 3—4 weeks. The rash is unilateral and confined to one or two adjacent dermatomes with a sharp cut off at or near the midline; this feature associated with the pain makes any other diagnosis unlikely. Pain may be continuous throughout this time and in the elderly may go on for months or even years.

Herpes zoster on the face is the result of involvement of the trigeminal nerve. With ophthalmic zoster the rash extends from the upper eyelid to the vertex of the skull; if vesicles occur on the side of the nose (nasocillary branch) the eye is likely to be involved and the patient should be referred to an ophthalmic surgeon.

## PHYTOPHOTODERMATITIS

This is due to plant juices containing photoactive chemicals (usually psoralens) being accidentally deposited on the skin, and causing an irritant dermatitis. Giant hogweed, rue, mustard and St John's wort are often responsible. The patient gives a history of having been in the garden clearing weeds, often using a strimmer, or

walking in the countryside on a sunny day. The rash is characteristically linear made up of blisters where the plants have touched the skin.

## CONTACT ALLERGIC ECZEMA

Linear blisters on the front of the wrist is characteristically due to the indoor primula (*Primula obconica*). Linear acute eczema elsewhere is usually due to some medicament such as a suntan lotion which has run down the skin.

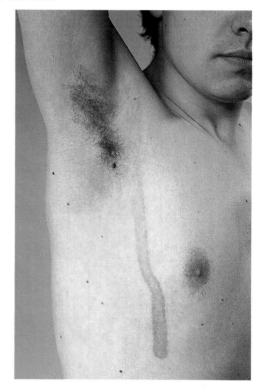

**3.16** Phytophotodermatitis due to Bergasol suntan lotion containing a psoralen; it has been applied to the arms and run down the front of the chest.

**3.15** Primula obconica plant.

**Face**
**Acute erythematous rash/lesions**
**Blisters/exudate/crusts**
**2 Widespread (most of face)**

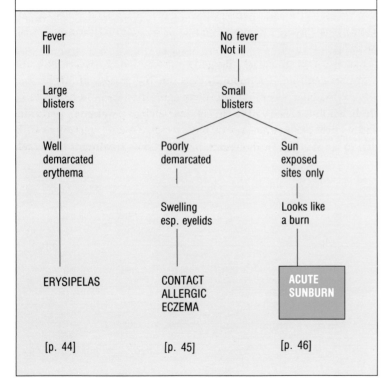

than not the site of entry is not obvious. The patient is un-well with fever, rigors and general malaise. The rash itself is bright red, well demarcated and may or may not contain large blisters in the centre. There is no associated lymphangitis or lymphadenopathy.

It is not usually possible to culture the organism from the skin and the measurement of the ASO titre is not helpful. Diagnosis is made on the characteristic clinical picture.

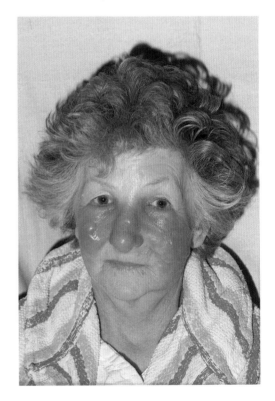

**3.17** Erysipelas.

## ERYSIPELAS

This is an acute, rapidly spreading rash caused by the entry into the skin of a group A beta-haemolytic streptococcus. More often

## ACUTE CONTACT ALLERGIC ECZEMA

An acute eczematous rash with vesicles, weeping and crusting is usually due to a contact allergic eczema. The onset of the rash is sudden with a poorly defined erythema, followed by swelling of the skin and blistering. If the eyelids are involved it may not be possible to open the eyes. It is usually symmetrical, and uncomfortable and itchy rather than painful as in herpes zoster.

There is no associated fever as in erysipelas.

Acute contact allergic eczema of the face is not usually due to cosmetics, but to an airborne allergen or an allergen in a cream applied to the face. The exact pattern of the rash depends on the allergen responsible. Airborne allergens cause a symmetrical eczema especially affecting the eyelids and cheeks, while allergens in medicaments only involve areas where these have been applied. Thus contact allergy to eyedrops results in conjunctivitis and eyelid involvement.

Examples of airborne allergens include sawdust, cement dust and phosphorous sesquisulphide from the smoke of 'strike anywhere' matches. Applied allergens contained in medicaments include lanolin, preservatives in creams (such as parabens), perfumes, and topical antihistamines or antibiotics. Severe reactions can be due to an allergen in the cream prescribed as treatment for a rash.

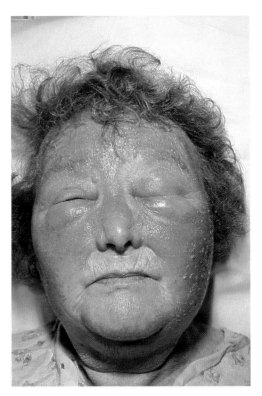

**3.18** Acute contact allergic eczema due to lanolin in a moisturising cream.

## ACUTE SUNBURN

Acute sunburn may result in pain, erythema and blisters on the skin and swelling of the eyelids. Usually the cause will be obvious, as the patient will have been exposed to strong sunlight. Other exposed areas will also be burnt.

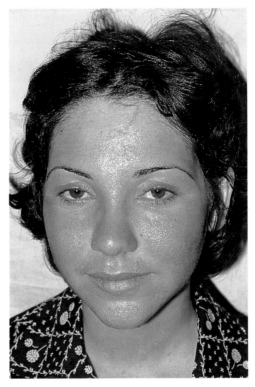

3.20 Acute sunburn: erythema and vesicles.

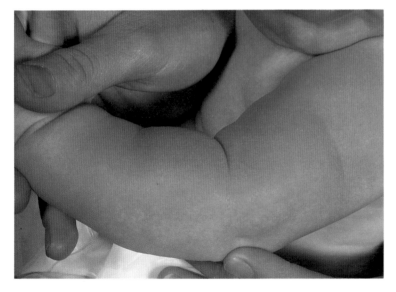

3.19 Acute sunburn in a 7 month old baby. Erythema and oedema but no vesicles.

## CHRONIC

**Face**
**Chronic erythematous rash/lesions**
**Normal surface**
**Macules and patches**

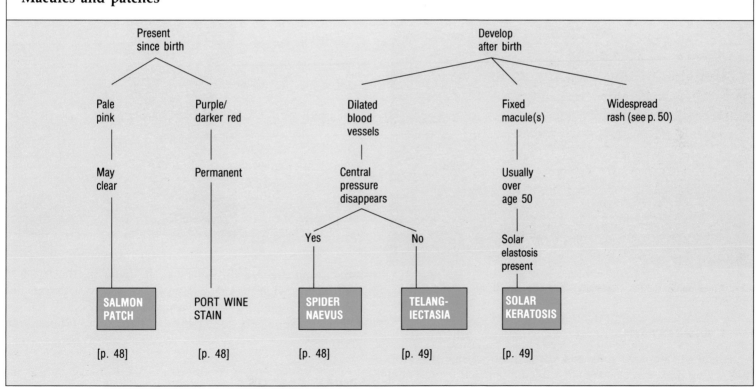

Present since birth

Develop after birth

Pale pink — May clear — **SALMON PATCH** — [p. 48]

Purple/ darker red — Permanent — PORT WINE STAIN — [p. 48]

Dilated blood vessels — Central pressure disappears
- Yes — **SPIDER NAEVUS** — [p. 48]
- No — **TELANG-IECTASIA** — [p. 49]

Fixed macule(s) — Usually over age 50 — Solar elastosis present — **SOLAR KERATOSIS** — [p. 49]

Widespread rash (see p. 50)

## SALMON PATCH

This is a pale pink patch, present at birth situated on the nape of the neck, forehead or eyelid. Pressure over the area will cause blanching, showing that it is due to dilated blood vessels. Those on the face usually disappear during the first year of life; those found on the nape of the neck do not, and usually persist throughout life.

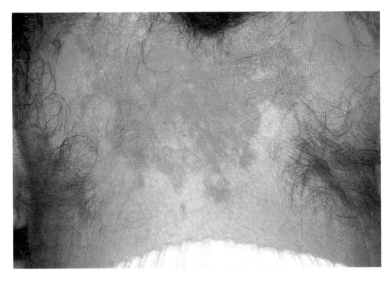

**3.21** Salmon patch (capillary haemangioma) on occipital area.

## PORT WINE STAIN

A permanent, more obvious and cosmetically disfiguring birth mark, being darker in colour than a salmon patch. It is present at birth and increases in size in proportion with growth. Port wine stains are very variable in size and colour (pink to deep red-

**3.22** Port wine stain.

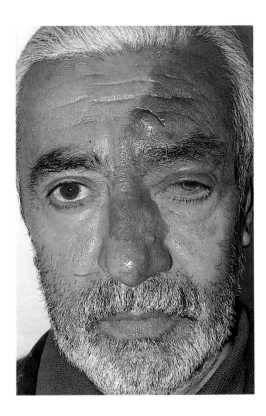

purple), and are usually unilateral. If involving the trigeminal area, the port wine stain may rarely be associated with ocular and intracranial angiomas, sometimes resulting in blindness, focal epilepsy, hemiplegia or mental retardation (Sturge-Weber syndrome).

## SPIDER NAEVUS

A single feeding central blood vessel (arteriole) with peripheral

**3.23** Spider naevus on tip of nose in a 4-year-old girl.

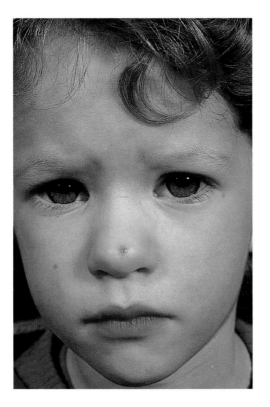

on the face due to weathering and may be associated with rosacea, scleroderma, or the application of potent topical steroids.

## SOLAR KERATOSIS

This may present as an area of fixed erythema on the face of a middle aged or elderly fair-skinned individual who has had a lot of sun exposure in the past (see p. 64).

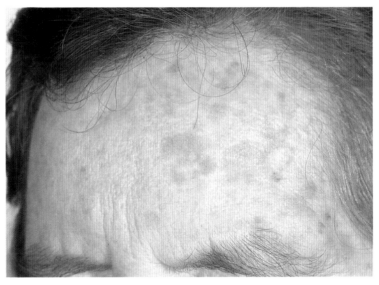

**3.24** Multiple solar keratoses on the forehead. These are often misdiagnosed: the key to the correct diagnosis is to feel the surface which is always rough.

radiating arms. Pressure (use a paper clip) on the central vessel results in obliteration of the lesion. Single naevi are extremely common in children. Larger numbers occur in pregnancy and in association with chronic liver disease.

## TELANGIECTASIA

A small area of visibly dilated blood vessels where there is no central vessel feeding it is called telangiectasia. It is very common

**Face**
**Chronic erythematous lesions/rash**
**Normal/smooth surface**
**Papules/plaques/nodules—Pustules not present (pustules present see p. 57)**
**1  Single/few (1–5) lesions**
    **a. No recent increase in size: see Chapter 4 p. 87; Chapter 5 p. 156**
    **b. Recent increase in size: see Chapter 5 p. 158**
**2  Multiple/widespread lesions/rash**

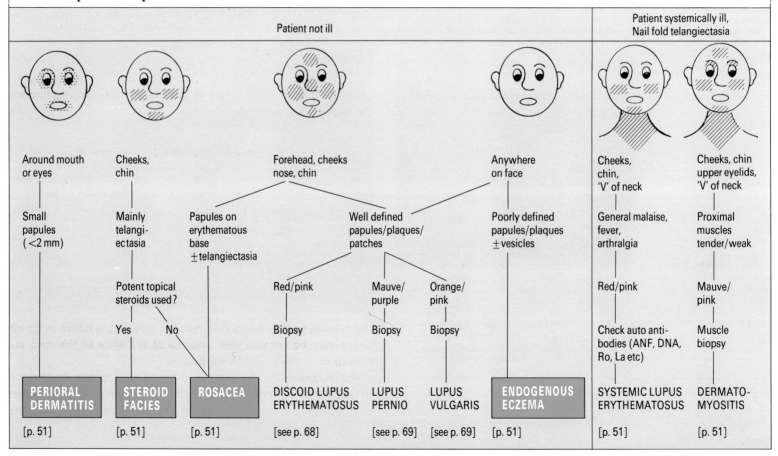

| Patient not ill | | | | | Patient systemically ill, Nail fold telangiectasia | |

Patient not ill:

| Around mouth or eyes | Cheeks, chin | Forehead, cheeks nose, chin | | | Anywhere on face | Cheeks, chin, 'V' of neck | Cheeks, chin upper eyelids, 'V' of neck |
|---|---|---|---|---|---|---|---|
| Small papules (<2 mm) | Mainly telangiectasia | Papules on erythematous base ±telangiectasia | Well defined papules/plaques/patches | | Poorly defined papules/plaques ±vesicles | General malaise, fever, arthralgia | Proximal muscles tender/weak |
| | Potent topical steroids used? | | | | | | |
| | Yes   No | | Red/pink  Mauve/purple  Orange/pink | | | Red/pink | Mauve/pink |
| | | | Biopsy   Biopsy   Biopsy | | | Check auto antibodies (ANF, DNA, Ro, La etc) | Muscle biopsy |
| **PERIORAL DERMATITIS** | **STEROID FACIES** | **ROSACEA** | DISCOID LUPUS ERYTHEMATOSUS  LUPUS PERNIO  LUPUS VULGARIS | | **ENDOGENOUS ECZEMA** | SYSTEMIC LUPUS ERYTHEMATOSUS | DERMATO-MYOSITIS |
| [p. 51] | [p. 51] | [p. 51] | [see p. 68]  [see p. 69]  [see p. 69] | | [p. 51] | [p. 51] | [p. 51] |

## ENDOGENOUS ECZEMA

Eczema should always be considered in the differential diagnosis since it is very common, but if looked for there should be some evidence of scaling (see p. 103).

## ROSACEA

Pustules do not necessarily have to be present in rosacea. The association of papules on red background in the characteristic

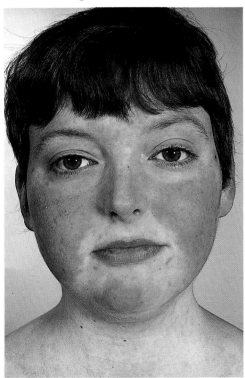

**3.25** Systemic lupus erythematosus in a 15-year-old boy: erythema but no scaling.

sites — cheeks, tip of nose, forehead and chin is typical (see p. 58).

## PERIORAL DERMATITIS

Perioral dermatitis should be considered in *young adults* where there are very small papules situated around the mouth, and who may have applied potent topical steroids to the face (see p. 60).

## STEROID FACIES

Telangiectasia on the cheeks and chin may follow the application of potent topical steroids to the face, particularly in patients over the age of 25 (see p. 59).

## SYSTEMIC LUPUS ERYTHEMATOSUS (SLE)

Red patches and plaques on sun exposed areas associated with fever and arthralgia are suggestive of SLE. Although the sites may be similar to rosacea, there are no papules or pustules. A positive antinuclear factor will confirm the diagnosis.

## DERMATOMYOSITIS

Weakness and tenderness of proximal muscles associated with a mauve or pink rash on the face, 'V' of the neck or in lines along the dorsum of the fingers and over the metacarpal bones is typical. There may be considerable oedema at the sites of the rash and dilatation of the nail fold capillaries.

The diagnosis can be confirmed by measuring muscle enzymes (creatine kinase), muscle biopsy or electromyography. In patients over the age of 40, there may be an associated internal malignancy.

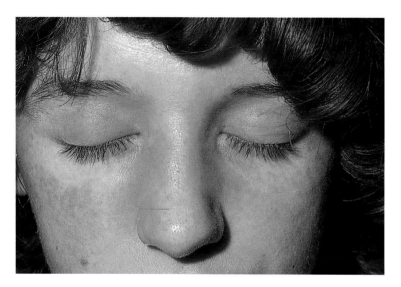

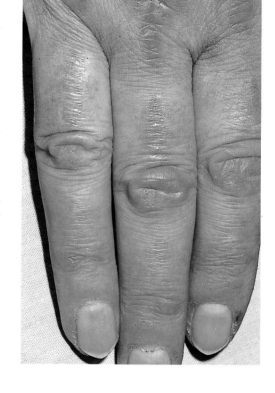

*Left*
**3.26** Dermatomyositis. The rash looks like SLE, but usually involves the eyelids as well as the cheeks.

*Right*
**3.27** Dermatomyositis: linear mauve plaques along the back of the fingers.

*Left below*
**3.28** Nail fold telangiectasia: found with SLE, dermatomyositis and systemic sclerosis.

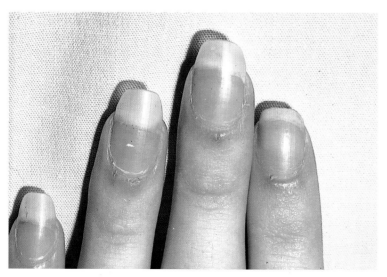

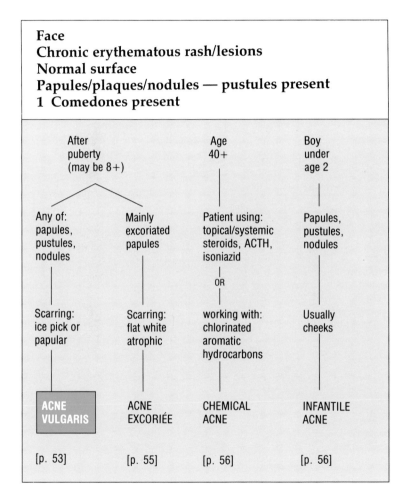

| After puberty (may be 8+) | | Age 40+ | Boy under age 2 |
|---|---|---|---|
| Any of: papules, pustules, nodules | Mainly excoriated papules | Patient using: topical/systemic steroids, ACTH, isoniazid OR | Papules, pustules, nodules |
| Scarring: ice pick or papular | Scarring: flat white atrophic | working with: chlorinated aromatic hydrocarbons | Usually cheeks |
| **ACNE VULGARIS** | ACNE EXCORIÉE | CHEMICAL ACNE | INFANTILE ACNE |
| [p. 53] | [p. 55] | [p. 56] | [p. 56] |

**Face
Chronic erythematous rash/lesions
Normal surface
Papules/plaques/nodules — pustules present
1 Comedones present**

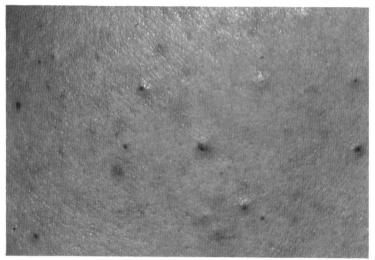

**3.29** Comedones: open and closed.

## ACNE VULGARIS

Acne is a disease of the sebaceous follicle. The hallmark of the disease is the comedone, a single blocked follicle. Everyone gets some acne. In girls it may appear several years before menstruation commences, sometimes as early as 8 years of age. In both sexes the peak incidence is 13–16 years, although it may continue into the 20s, 30s and occasionally later. Acne occurs on the face, chest and back depending on the distribution of the sebaceous follicles in that individual.

The factors involved in the aetiology are shown in Fig. 3.30. Genetic factors are important in determining the severity, duration and clinical pattern. There is no evidence that diet influences acne, and it is certainly not a result of over indulgence in chocolates, fatty or 'junk' food.

The evolution of acne lesions from a blocked sebaceous follicle is shown in Fig. 3.31. The black colour of open comedones is due to melanin, not dirt.

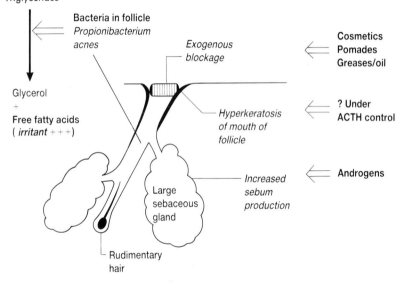

**3.30** Aetiology of acne.

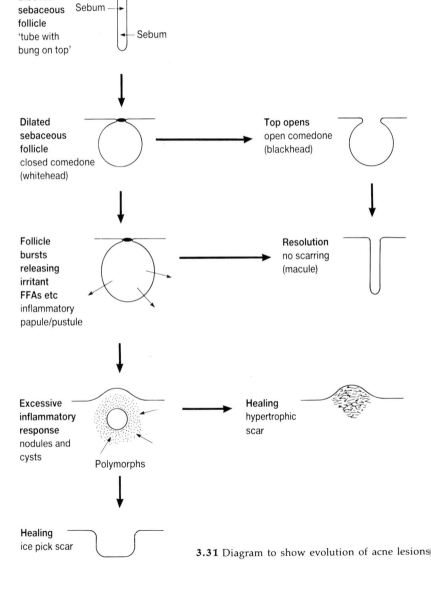

**3.31** Diagram to show evolution of acne lesions

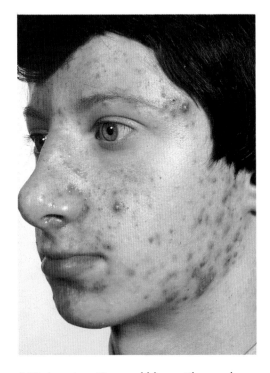

**3.32** Acne in a 15-year-old boy with comedones, papules and pustules.

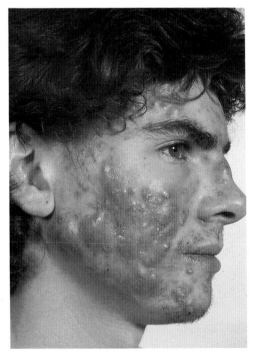

**3.33** Severe nodular acne in a 17-year-old boy.

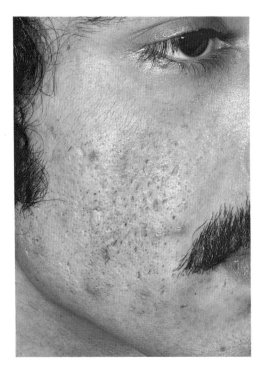

**3.34** Ice pick scars and papules on cheek.

The diagnosis is usually easy, but comedones must be present before it is made. Comedones, papules, pustules, nodules, cysts and scarring on the face or trunk of a young person is unique to acne, but occasionally folliculitis or even a papular form of eczema can mimic acne. Multiple epidermoid cysts may be confused with severe nodulo-cystic acne. Rosacea looks similar but affects an older population; there are no comedones, and the papules and pustules occur over a general erythematous background with telangiectasia.

## ACNE EXCORIÉE

This variety of acne occurs predominantly in women and most of the lesions are excoriated. Usually the degree of acne is mild, pustules are few or absent, and all the lesions have been scratched or picked. Round or oval white scars are the most obvious finding confirming that the condition is largely self induced.

## CHEMICAL AND DRUG INDUCED ACNE

A rash that looks like acne occurring at the wrong site or in the wrong age group should make one think of this possibility. Chlorinated aromatic hydrocarbons used in insecticides, fungicides and wood preservatives cause severe acne which may continue for years after exposure has ceased. Insoluble cutting oils, coal tars and corticosteroids may induce acne when applied topically to the skin; so can cosmetics, especially thick make up. A series of ingested medicaments may worsen acne or precipitate it. These include systemic steroids, ACTH, and isoniazid.

## INFANTILE ACNE

Acne is occasionally seen in infancy in boys. It is confined to the face, with comedones, papules, pustules and nodules. It usually disappears during the first 2 years of life and presumably is due to maternal androgens. It is not seen in girls.

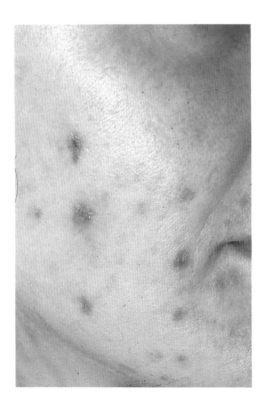

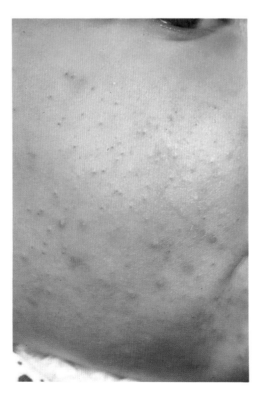

*Far left*
**3.35** Acne excoriée in a 23-year-old lady showing all the papules excoriated, no comedones and early scars.

*Left*
**3.36** Infantile acne in an 8 month-old boy with comedones, and occasional pustules and papules.

**Face**
**Chronic erythematous lesions/rash**
**Normal/smooth surface**
**Papules/plaques/nodules—Pustules present**
**2 Comedones absent**

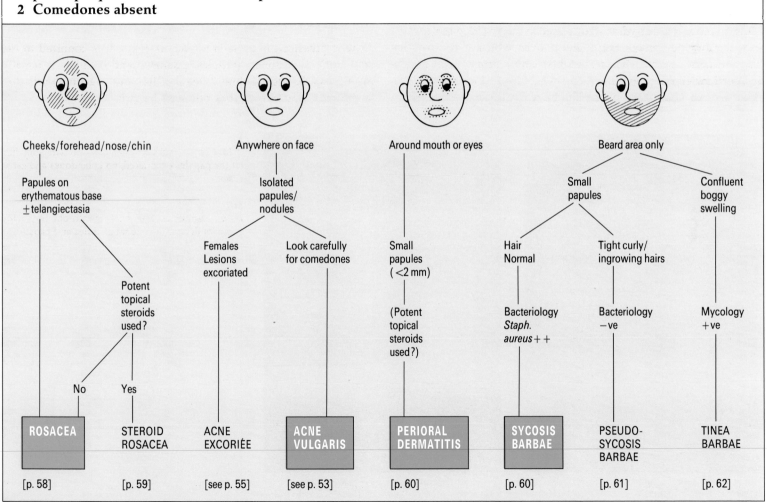

Cheeks/forehead/nose/chin

Papules on
erythematous base
±telangiectasia

Potent
topical
steroids
used?

No — **ROSACEA** [p. 58]

Yes — STEROID ROSACEA [p. 59]

Anywhere on face

Isolated
papules/
nodules

Females
Lesions
excoriated — ACNE EXCORIÉE [see p. 55]

Look carefully
for comedones — **ACNE VULGARIS** [see p. 53]

Around mouth or eyes

Small
papules
(<2 mm)

(Potent
topical
steroids
used?)

**PERIORAL DERMATITIS** [p. 60]

Beard area only

Small
papules

Hair
Normal

Bacteriology
*Staph.*
*aureus*++

**SYCOSIS BARBAE** [p. 60]

Tight curly/
ingrowing hairs

Bacteriology
−ve

PSEUDO-
SYCOSIS
BARBAE [p. 61]

Confluent
boggy
swelling

Mycology
+ve

TINEA
BARBAE [p. 62]

## ROSACEA

This is a rash which looks like acne but on a red background. Red patches (erythema and telangiectasia) occur on the cheeks, chin, forehead and tip of nose; in addition there are papules and pustules but no comedones. If the patient is undressed papules and pustules may be seen on the upper trunk too. Rosacea affects women more commonly than men, and the main incidence is over the age of 40, although it can occur at any age. Complications such as sore red eyes (blepharitis, conjunctivitis and keratitis), chronic lymphoedema of the face and rhinophyma occur more commonly in men.

Rosacea needs to be distinguished from acne, seborrhoeic eczema, perioral dermatitis and other, rare conditions resulting in facial erythema and papules. Acne occurs in a younger age group and there should be comedones present. Seborrhoeic eczema is scaly, there are no pustules and the naso-labial folds rather than cheeks are affected; scaling will also be present in the scalp and possibly elsewhere. Perioral dermatitis occurs in young adults, is

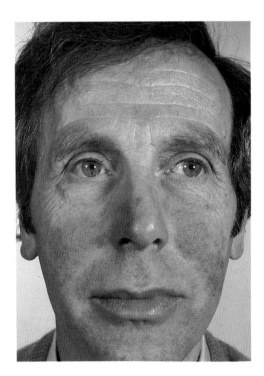
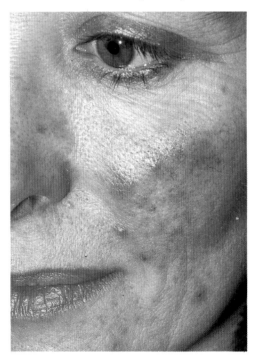
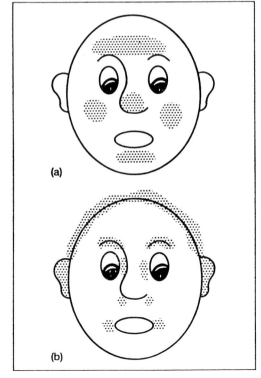

(a)

(b)

around the mouth only and the individual papules and pustules are very small. Systemic lupus erythematosus may be confused because of the redness of the face, but there are no papules or pustules and the patient is usually unwell.

## RHINOPHYMA

Enlargement of the skin of the nose due to hyperplasia of the sebaceous glands is called rhinophyma. It occurs in individuals who have rosacea. Contrary to popular belief it is not associated with excessive alcohol intake.

## STEROID ROSACEA

Application of potent topical fluorinated steroids to the face can result in a rosacea-like rash. Telangiectasia is the most obvious feature although small papules and pustules may also be present. It is reversible if the topical steroids are stopped.

*Facing page*
*Left*
**3.37** Rosacea: red plaques on cheeks and nose.

*Centre*
**3.38** Rosacea: close up to show telangiectasia, papules and pustules.

*Right*
**3.39** Distribution of (a) rosacea and (b) seborrhoeic eczema (see pp 65 & 106).

*Right*
**3.40** Rhinophyma.

*Far right*
**3.41** Steroid rosacea: note involvement of naso-labial folds, telangiectasia and small papules and pustules.

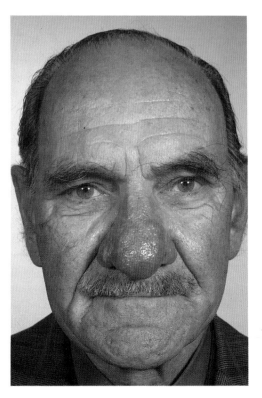

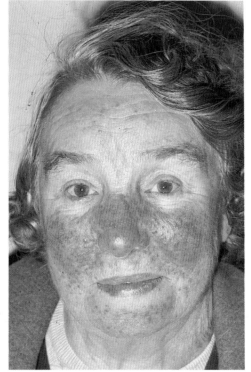

## PERIORAL DERMATITIS

Perioral dermatitis is a condition of young adults who have been applying potent topical corticosteroids to the face. Minute (1 mm) red papules and pustules appear around the mouth, typically sparing the skin immediately adjacent to the lips; occasionally it occurs around the eyes (periocular dermatitis). In some individuals there is no history of topical steroid use.

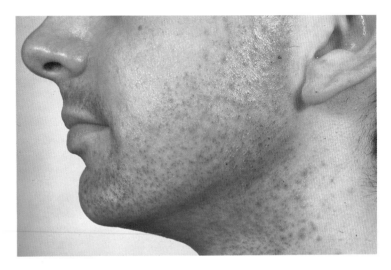

3.43 Sycosis barbae: follicular papules and pustules (tops removed by shaving).

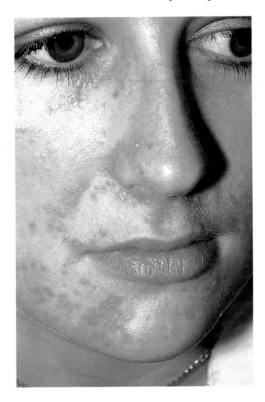

3.42 Perioral dermatitis.

## SYCOSIS BARBAE

This is folliculitis of the beard area caused by infection with *Staphylococcus aureus*. The trauma of shaving results in spread and innoculation of the bacteria over the beard area. The organism is often cultured from the nose, as well as the infected follicles.

Sycosis barbae only occurs in men who shave, and presents as follicular papules and pustules scattered over the beard area. The papules and pustules usually remain discrete, but if neighbouring follicules are involved more extensive areas of erythema, pustules and crusting can occur. The depth of infection varies but only in rare cases does destruction of the follicle and scarring occur. The hairs remain firmly attached so they cannot be plucked out easily, a feature that distinguishes bacterial from fungal infections.

Diagnosis is usually obvious, but may easily be confused with pseudo-sycosis barbae where ingrowing hairs produce inflammation.

## PSEUDO-SYCOSIS BARBAE

This condition is due to ingrowing hairs in the beard area. It is more common in Negroes with their naturally tight curly hair. The

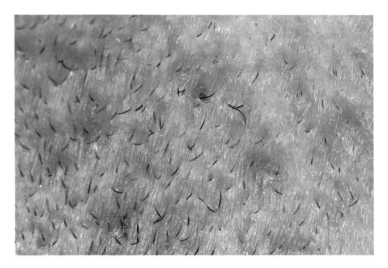

3.45 Pseudo-sycosis barbae: close up of ingrowing hairs (compare with Fig 3.43).

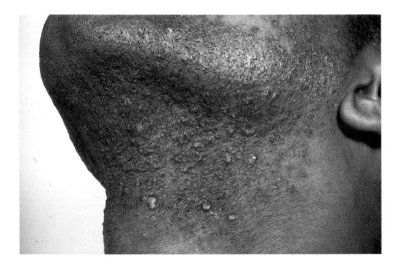

3.44 Pseudo-sycosis barbae in Negro: inflammatory papules at tip of curly hairs.

from the bacterial form where the lesion occurs at the mouth of the hair follicle as the hair emerges. It should be possible with a needle to extract the tip of the hair from the skin, although some hairs may be completely buried within a papule.

inflammatory papules and pustules are due to a foreign body reaction where the hair grows into the skin. This determines the site of the papules and pustules, and distinguishes the condition

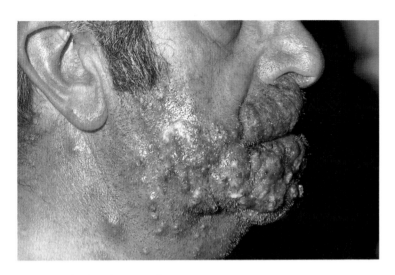

**3.46** Tinea barbae due to cattle ringworm.

## TINEA BARBAE

This uncommon infection is due to animal ringworm (usually *Trichophyton verrucosum*), and occurs commonly in farm workers. A confluent boggy swelling studded with multiple pustules occurs on the chin or cheek. The hairs come out easily and can be examined for fungi. Secondary infection with staphylococci can occur, so a positive bacterial culture may be misleading.

**Face**
**Chronic erythematous rash/lesions**
**Scaly surface**
**Multiple papules/plaques**
**1 Poorly defined border**

Scratch rash with nail. Palpate with finger tips

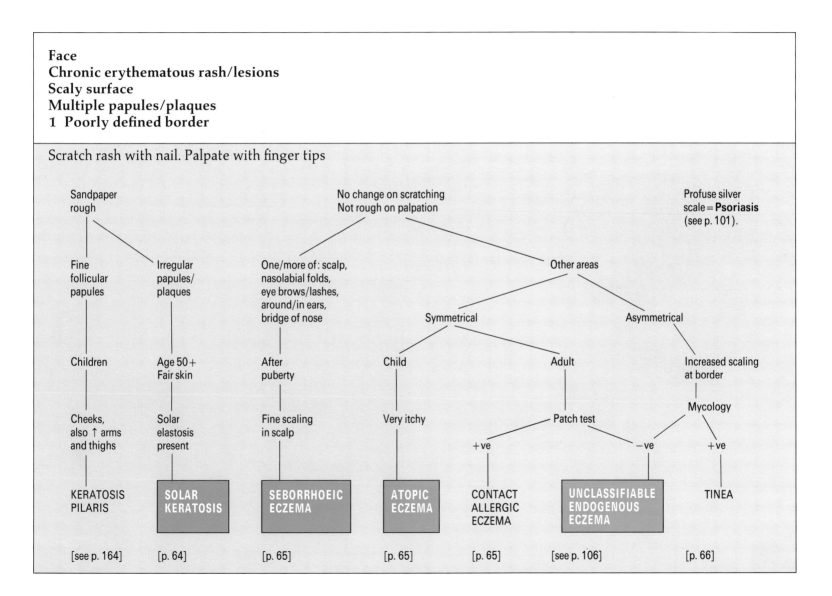

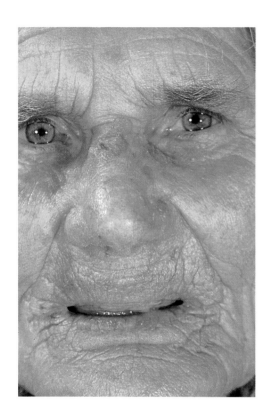

**3.47** Solar elastosis in a 74-year-old lady. Note the solar keratosis on the bridge of the nose.

## SOLAR KERATOSES

Widespread solar keratoses may be confused with eczema on the face. The 'scaling' due to accumulation of keratin on the surface feels like sandpaper.

The patients will probably be over 50, have fair skin (burn rather than tan on sun exposure) and blue eyes, and give a history of working out of doors or living abroad (20+ years ago). They will have **solar elastosis** as evidence of solar damage to the skin. This is a creamy-yellow discolouration of the skin with increased skin markings and follicular openings on the face, neck and (bald) scalp. These changes (wrinkles) are thought to be due to ageing, but in fact, it is the sun and not the passage of time that has caused the damage.

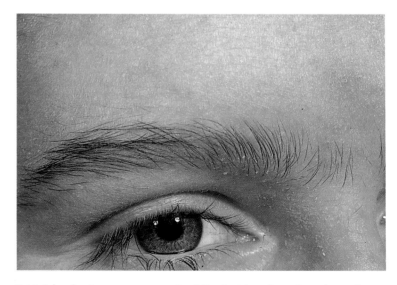

**3.48** Seborrhoeic eczema: a poorly defined pink scaly rash in the eyebrows and adjacent skin.

## ECZEMA ON THE FACE

The most likely cause of poorly defined scaly plaques on the face is chronic eczema. The distribution and age of the patient determine the type of eczema. Eczema confined to the face may be due to contact allergy (see p. 45) which can be confirmed or refuted by patch testing, see p. 11.

*Atopic eczema*
This is the commonest type in young children, but may continue into or re-occur in adult life, see p. 103.

*Seborrhoeic eczema*
In adults scaling around the sides of the nose, in the eyelashes and eyebrows, and in front, behind or in the ear is due to seborrhoeic eczema: fine scaling in the scalp confirms this diagnosis, see p. 106.

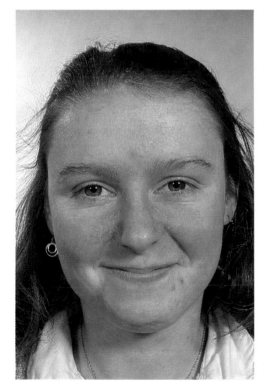

**3.49** Seborrhoeic eczema affecting the nasolabial folds.

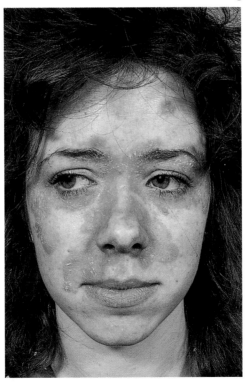

**3.50** Psoriasis on the face (compare with Fig 3.49.).

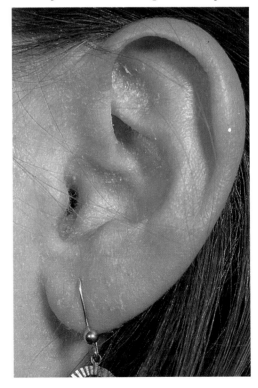

**3.51** Seborrhoeic eczema: scaling in the external ear.

## TINEA (RINGWORM)

Although frequently diagnosed in general practice, ringworm is uncommon on the face. It should be suspected if a red scaly rash is *unilateral* or very much more on one side than the other. It may have a ringed appearance with relatively normal skin in the centre with a raised pink scaly edge, or be poorly defined. Common rashes such as eczema and psoriasis may also be annular. All unilateral rashes should therefore be scraped, and the scale sent off for mycology culture (see p. 9).

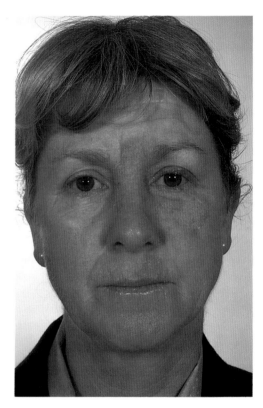

**3.53** Tinea on the face: suspect in any unilateral red scaly rash

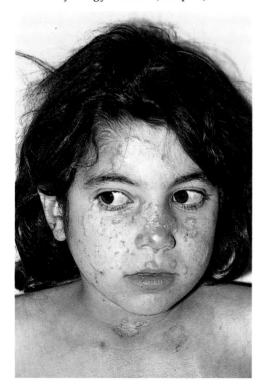

**3.52** Tinea on the face: a red scaly rash much more on the right than the left, although not in a ring.

**Face**
**Chronic erythematous rash/lesions**
**Scaly surface**
**Multiple/widespread papules/plaques**
**2  Well defined border**

Scratch rash with nail. Look at colour

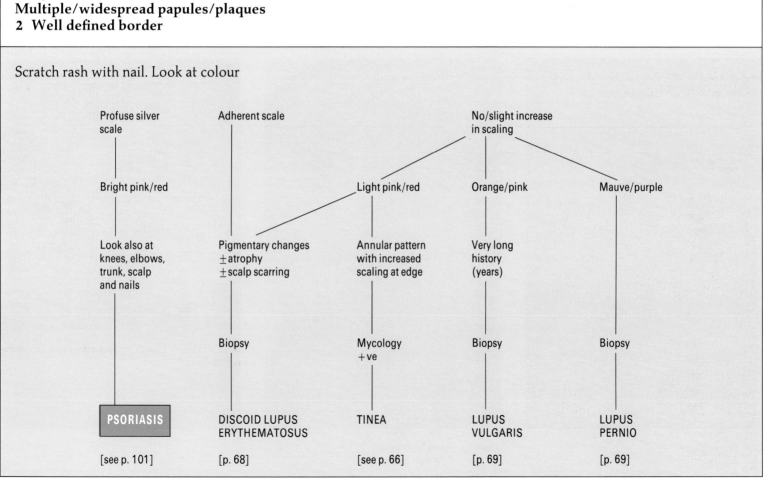

Profuse silver scale → Bright pink/red → Look also at knees, elbows, trunk, scalp and nails → **PSORIASIS** [see p. 101]

Adherent scale → Pigmentary changes ±atrophy ±scalp scarring → Biopsy → DISCOID LUPUS ERYTHEMATOSUS [p. 68]

No/slight increase in scaling:

Light pink/red → Annular pattern with increased scaling at edge → Mycology +ve → TINEA [see p. 66]

Orange/pink → Very long history (years) → Biopsy → LUPUS VULGARIS [p. 69]

Mauve/purple → Biopsy → LUPUS PERNIO [p. 69]

## DISCOID LUPUS ERYTHEMATOSUS (DLE)

A benign form of lupus erythematosus where the skin is involved without any systemic illness. Females are more commonly affected than males, and DLE usually occurs between the ages of 25 and 40.

Well-defined red scaly plaques occur on the face and scalp, and may be precipitated by sunlight. The scale is quite different from that occuring in psoriasis or eczema; it does not produce the silver scaling on scratching, and is more rough and adherent than that of eczema. Often the scale plugs the hair follicles so on removal looks like 'carpet tacking'. There may be both atrophy and pigment change (both hypo- and hyperpigmentation).

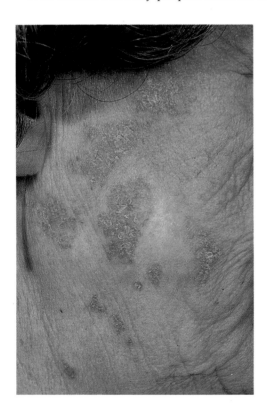

3.54 Discoid lupus erythematosus.

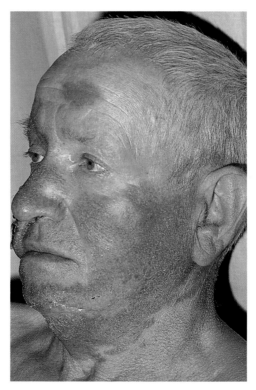

3.55 Lupus vulgaris. This orangy-pink plaque had been present for > 50 years, gradually extending. It had always been assumed to be a birth mark!

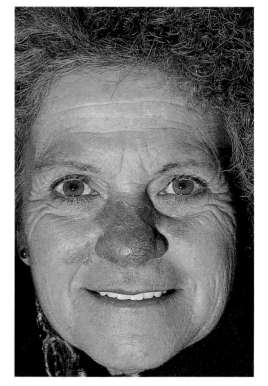

3.56 Lupus pernio (sarcoidosis) on the nose.

The diagnosis should only be considered when more common causes of scaling on the face are excluded. The appearance is characteristic, however, and can be confirmed by skin biopsy.

## LUPUS VULGARIS

This is even rarer than discoid lupus erythematosus, and is a chronic tuberculous infection of the dermis. A slowly enlarging orangy-pink plaque is typical, which may even be misdiagnosed as a birth mark! A biopsy is needed to confirm the diagnosis.

## LUPUS PERNIO

This is an unusual skin manifestation of sarcoidosis. A chronic purple plaque occurs on the face, most characteristically on the cheeks or nose.

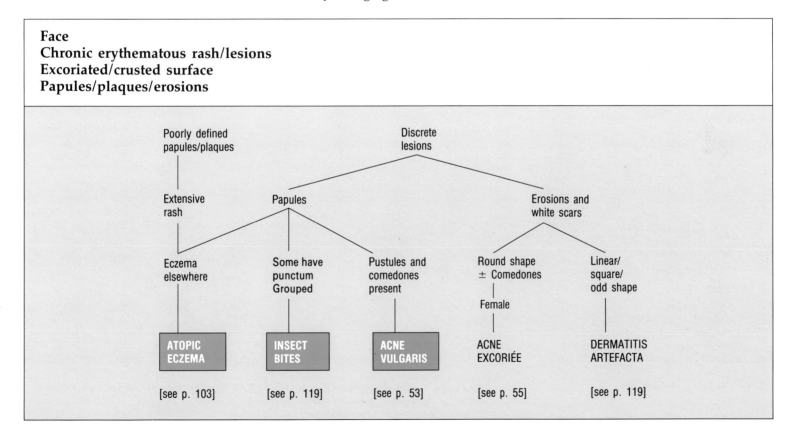

**Face
Chronic erythematous rash/lesions
Excoriated/crusted surface
Papules/plaques/erosions**

Poorly defined papules/plaques

Discrete lesions

Extensive rash

Papules

Erosions and white scars

Eczema elsewhere

Some have punctum Grouped

Pustules and comedones present

Round shape ± Comedones

Linear/ square/ odd shape

Female

**ATOPIC ECZEMA**

**INSECT BITES**

**ACNE VULGARIS**

ACNE EXCORIÉE

DERMATITIS ARTEFACTA

[see p. 103]

[see p. 119]

[see p. 53]

[see p. 55]

[see p. 119]

# Chapter 4
# Erythematous Rashes and Lesions on Trunk and Limbs*

**ACUTE** ( <2 weeks duration)

**Normal surface**
Transient lesions, 72
Maculo-papular rash, 74
Papules/nodules – NO PUSTULES
   few lesions, 77
   multiple/widespread lesions, 78
Pustules, 79

**Blisters/crust/exudate/erosion**
Localized, see Chapter 3 p. 39
Widespread, 81

**Generalized rash,** 82

**CHRONIC** ( >2 weeks duration)

**Normal surface**
Macules/patches, 85
Papules/plaques/nodules
  PUSTULES NEVER PRESENT
  single or few (1–5) lesions
    small papules ( <0.5cm), 87
    larger papules ( >0.5cm)/plaques/nodules, 88
  widespread/multiple lesions/rash
    small papules ( <0.5cm), 92
    larger papules ( >0.5cm)/plaques/nodules, 93
  PUSTULES PRESENT, 96

**Scaly surface**
Single/few papules/plaques, 97
Nodules, see p. 167
Multiple lesions/rash
  some lesions >2cm size, 100
    chronic eczema, 102
  all lesions <2cm size, 108
Generalized rash/itching ( >50% body), 113

**Excoriated surface** (intense itching), 115

**Crusted/ulcerated/eroded surface**
Single/few papules/plaques/nodules, 121

**Crusts/erosions/blisters**
Widespread/multiple lesions/rash, 122

***For lower legs see Chapter 7 p. 185 and for dorsum of forearm Chapter 8 p. 205.**

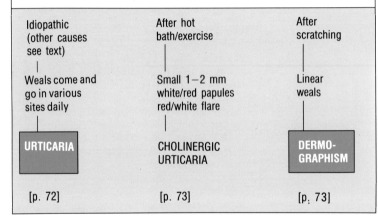

**Trunk and limbs**
**Acute erythematous rash/lesions**
**Normal surface**
**Transient patches/papules/plaques**

Transient lesions last in any one site for less than 24 hours, although lesions may be present continuously at different sites. If in doubt, draw around lesion and see if it has moved by the next day.

| Idiopathic (other causes see text) | After hot bath/exercise | After scratching |
|---|---|---|
| Weals come and go in various sites daily | Small 1–2 mm white/red papules red/white flare | Linear weals |
| **URICARIA** | CHOLINERGIC URTICARIA | **DERMO-GRAPHISM** |
| [p. 72] | [p. 73] | [p. 73] |

## URTICARIA

This is the commonest rash where individual lesions come and go within a few hours. A central itchy white papule or plaque due to dermal oedema (weal) is surrounded by an erythematous flare (like Lewis's triple response). The lesions are variable in size and shape, and may be associated with swelling of the soft tissues of the eyelids, lips and tongue (angio-oedema).

Urticaria is thought to be due to release of histamine and other mediators from mast cells in the skin; why this occurs is not always understood.

**Urticarial vasculitis** occurs if individual lesions last for longer than 24 hours since the histology and causes are different.

### Acute urticaria

This is a type I allergic response and occurs within a few minutes of contact with an allergen either on the skin (e.g. nettle rash), or ingested (e.g. strawberries or penicillin). The rash disappears spontaneously within an hour. Contact with the same allergen again will result in a further episode.

### Chronic urticaria

Here the weals come and go over a period of months or years. Individual lesions always last less than 24 hours, new lesions appearing daily or every few days. It can occur at any time of day or night and is not a type I allergic response.

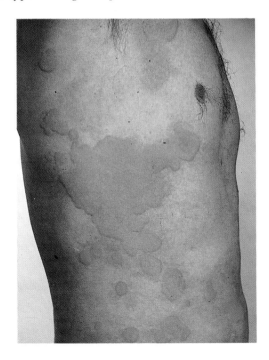

4.1 Urticaria.

Possible causes of chronic urticaria are as follows.

1 Psychological factors:
 ongoing stressful situations
 very hectic lifestyle
 guilt

2 Drugs such as aspirin, codeine and opiates. These have a direct degranulating effect on mast cells, and are the commonest cause of infrequent episodes of urticaria, e.g. when the patient has a cold and takes medicines containing aspirin.

3 Food additives such as tartrazines, benzoates etc, which are chemically similar to aspirin

4 Chronic infections and infestations:
 bacterial (sinus, dental, chest, gall bladder)
 fungal (candidiasis)
 intestinal worms

5 General medical conditions — hyperthyroidism, chronic active hepatitis, SLE.

6 Idiopathic — no cause can be found

## CHOLINERGIC URTICARIA

Small red papules (1–3 mm diameter) surrounded by an area of vasoconstriction occur after exercise or hot baths, mainly in young adults. The diagnosis can easily be confirmed if the lesions are not present by making the patient exercise vigorously for a few minutes.

## DERMOGRAPHISM

About 5% percent of the population produce a triple response in the skin after scratching or other minor trauma, and these patients will often complain of itching. Fortunately it tends to get better spontaneously after months or occasionally years.

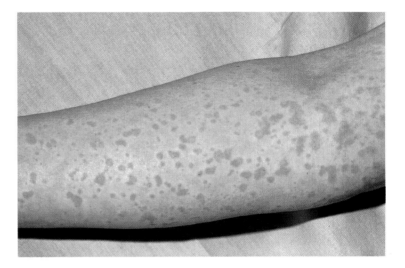

4.2 Cholinergic urticaria.

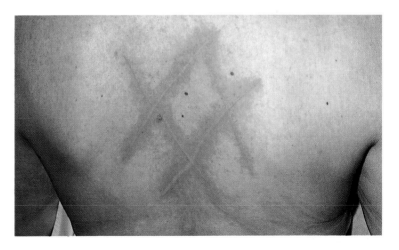

4.3 Dermographism.

**Acute erythematous maculo-papular rashes—face, trunk and limbs—normal surface**
Small red macules and papules which coalesce to become confluent. Scaling does not occur, which distinguishes this type of rash from others such as guttate psoriasis (see p. 109) or pityriasis rosea (see p. 111). Secondary scaling and purpura can occur if the eruption is very severe.

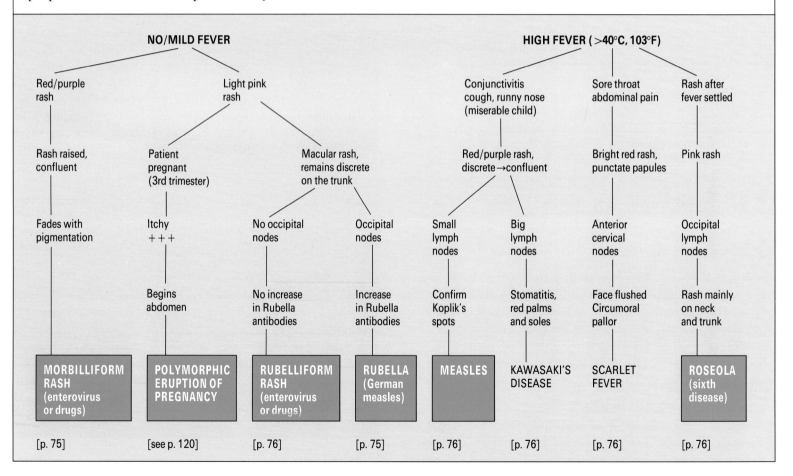

## MORBILLIFORM RASH

This is a rash that looks like measles but has no prodromal symptoms. It is usually due to an enterovirus (ECHO or Cocksackie) or a drug (e.g. ampicillin). It gets better spontaneously over 1–2 weeks and needs no treatment.

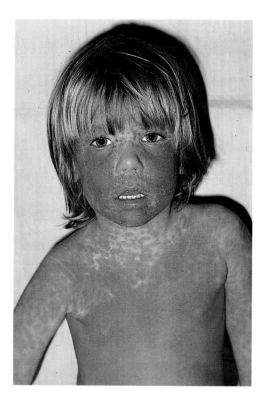

**4.4** Morbilliform eruption in a 2 year old boy.

## RUBELLA (GERMAN MEASLES)

Rubella is a viral illness spread by inhalation of infected droplets. After an incubation period of 14–21 days, the rash appears. Discrete macules occur on the face or neck, and rapidly spread to the trunk and limbs over about 24 hours. They usually remain discrete, but may become confluent. After 24 hours the rash begins to disappear, initially from the face and then from the trunk and limbs. It is often associated with enlarged occipital and posterior cervical lymph nodes, and sometimes an arthritis.

If the diagnosis is suspected, rubella antibody titres should be measured immediately and after 10 days so that the diagnosis can be confirmed. Many other viral infections look like rubella but do not carry the same risk to pregnant mothers (cataracts, nerve deafness and cardiac abnormalities in the foetus if infection occurs in the first trimester).

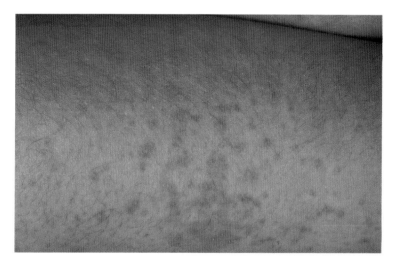

**4.5** Rubella.

## RUBELLIFORM AND ROSEOLIFORM RASHES

Probably more than 50 percent of rashes that look like rubella are in fact due to enteroviruses. Occipital nodes may even be enlarged making this an unreliable diagnostic feature.

## MEASLES

After an incubation period of about 10 days, the child becomes miserable with a high fever, runny nose, conjunctivitis, photophobia, brassy cough and inflamed tonsils. Koplik spots on the buccal mucosa are diagnostic at this stage (look like grains of salt on a red base). On day 4 of the illness a red macular rash appears behind the ears and spreads onto the face, trunk and limbs. The macules may become papules, which join together to become confluent. It lasts up to 10 days leaving brown pigmentation and some scaling.

## KAWASAKI'S DISEASE (MUCOCUTANEOUS LYMPH NODE SYNDROME)

This disease may be confused with measles, but must be recognized because of the potentially serious associated myocarditis. It occurs in young children under the age of 5 (50 percent under 2 years of age). The onset is acute with fever, red eyes, dry lips and prominent papillae on the tongue. The most characteristic signs are the large glands in the neck, the rash on the trunk and limbs, and red palms and soles which later peel.

*γ Globulin + Aspirin*

## SCARLET FEVER

Scarlet fever is due to a beta haemolytic streptococcus which produces an erythrogenic toxin. The condition seems to be less common than it used to be. After an incubation period of 2—5 days there is a sudden fever, with anorexia and sore throat. The tonsils are swollen with a white exudate, and there is painful lymphadenopathy in the neck. The tongue is furred initially, but later becomes red with prominent papillae (strawberry tongue). The rash appears on the second day as a widespread punctate erythema which rapidly becomes confluent. The face is flushed except for circumoral pallor. After about a week the rash fades followed by peeling of the skin. *Streptococcus pyogenes* can be grown from the throat and the ASOT is raised.

## ROSEOLA INFANTUM (SIXTH DISEASE)

This is the commonest rash of this kind in children under the age of 2. The rash is preceded by a high fever but the child remains well. After 3—5 days the fever goes and the rash, which looks like rubella, appears on the trunk. It lasts only 1—2 days and then disappears.

**Trunk, limbs, face**
**Acute erythematous lesions**
**Normal surface**
**Single/few (1—5) isolated papules/nodules**

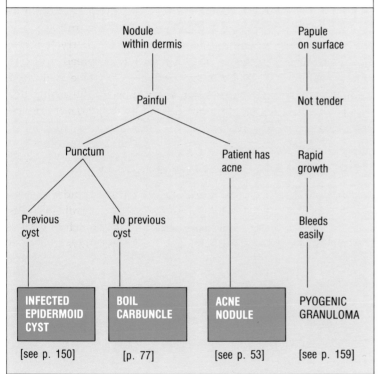

## BOIL AND CARBUNCLE

A boil is an abscess of a single hair follicle (Figs. 4.6, 4.9) caused by *Staphylococcus aureus* which may also be isolated from the nose or perineum. Single or multiple tender red nodules with a central punctum can occur anywhere on the body except the palms or soles. Without treatment the pus will point onto the surface and be discharged leaving a scar.

An abscess of several adjacent hair follicles is called a carbuncle. It looks just like a boil but is larger and has several openings onto the surface.

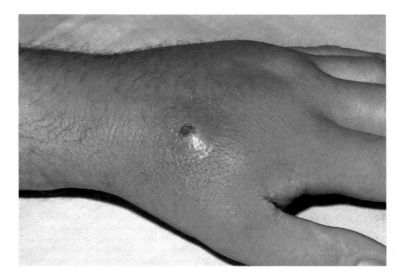

**4.6** Boil on back of hand.

**Trunk and limbs**
**Acute erythematous rash**
**Normal/smooth surface**
**Widespread/multiple papules and plaques—No pustules present**

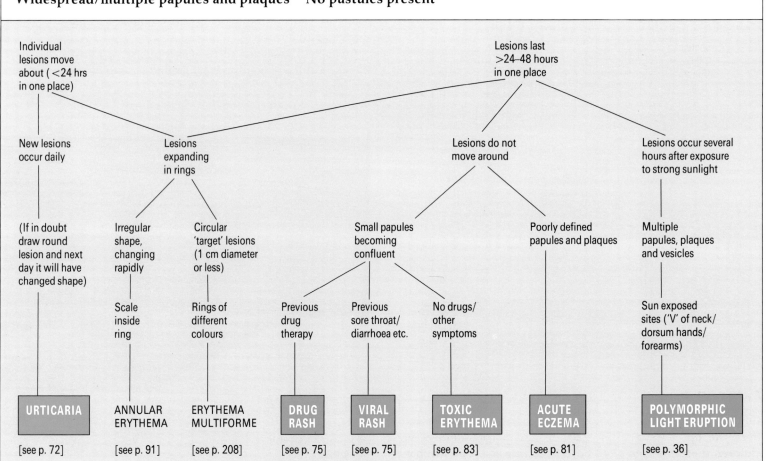

Individual lesions move about ( <24 hrs in one place)

Lesions last >24–48 hours in one place

New lesions occur daily

Lesions expanding in rings

Lesions do not move around

Lesions occur several hours after exposure to strong sunlight

(If in doubt draw round lesion and next day it will have changed shape)

Irregular shape, changing rapidly

Circular 'target' lesions (1 cm diameter or less)

Small papules becoming confluent

Poorly defined papules and plaques

Multiple papules, plaques and vesicles

Scale inside ring

Rings of different colours

Previous drug therapy

Previous sore throat/ diarrhoea etc.

No drugs/ other symptoms

Sun exposed sites ('V' of neck/ dorsum hands/ forearms)

| **URTICARIA** | ANNULAR ERYTHEMA | ERYTHEMA MULTIFORME | **DRUG RASH** | **VIRAL RASH** | **TOXIC ERYTHEMA** | **ACUTE ECZEMA** | **POLYMORPHIC LIGHT ERUPTION** |

[see p. 72]   [see p. 91]   [see p. 208]   [see p. 75]   [see p. 75]   [see p. 83]   [see p. 81]   [see p. 36]

**Trunk, limbs, face**
**Acute erythematous rash/lesions**
**Normal surface**
**Pustules**

Widespread pustules Intervening skin normal

Pustules on scaly/ erythematous skin

Face and trunk — Follicular lesions

Eczema present — Shallow pustules ? Previous psoriasis

Papules, vesicles and crusts

Legs, buttocks

Follicular pustules

Patient unwell/ fever

| CHICKEN POX (Varicella) | FOLLICULITIS | ECZEMA WITH FOLLICULITIS | GENERALIZED PUSTULAR PSORIASIS |
|---|---|---|---|
| [p. 79] | [p. 80] | [p. 80] | [see p. 84] |

period is usually 14–15 days, and patients are infectious from the day before to 7 days after the rash appears.

The prodromal illness is usually mild, so that the rash is the first evidence of illness. The lesions start off as pink macules, which develop quickly into papules, tense vesicles, pustules and then crusts. Crops of lesions occur over a few days so that there are always lesions at different stages of development present. These are very itchy and secondary infection may lead to pock-like scarring. Typically it occurs on the face and trunk rather than the limbs.

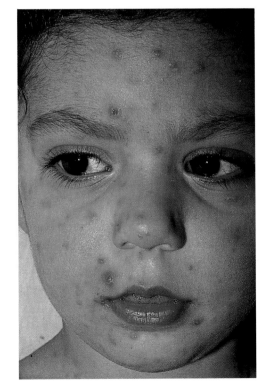

4.7 Chicken pox: note the presence of macules, papules, vesicles and pustules all at the same time.

## CHICKEN POX (HERPES VARICELLA-ZOSTER)

Chicken pox is a highly infectious illness spread by droplet infection from the upper respiratory tract. In urban communities most children under the age of 10 have been infected. The incubation

## FOLLICULITIS

Superficial infection of hair follicles is very common. A small bead of pus sits around a protruding hair, and there may be slight erythema at the base. One or several follicles may be involved, but there is no tenderness or involvement of the deep part of the follicle. It is usually due to *Staphylococcus aureus* which may be carried in the patient's nose or perineum. It can be made worse, or be caused by, the application of greasy ointments to the skin, tar preparations or elastoplast. The wearing of oily overalls may precipitate folliculitis of the thighs (oil acne) with plugged follicles and pustules.

## ECZEMA WITH FOLLICULITIS

Patients with eczema are particularly susceptible to developing folliculitis, mainly because of the application of greasy ointments. Changing the treatment to a cream may help.

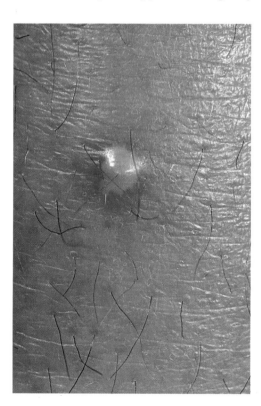

**4.8** Folliculitis: pustule with a hair in the centre.

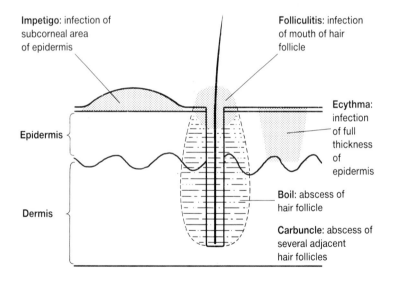

**4.9** Site of involvement of staphylococcal infections in the skin.

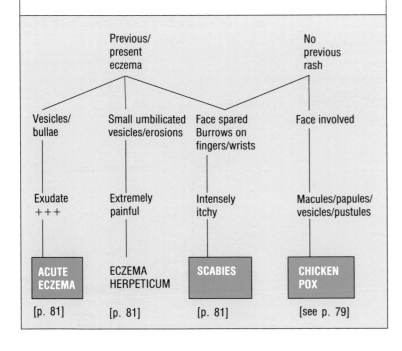

**Trunk and limbs**
**Acute erythematous rash/lesions**
**Blisters, crusts, erosions**
**1  Localized lesions (see Chapter 3 p. 39)**
**2  Widespread rash/lesions**

Previous/present eczema — No previous rash

Vesicles/bullae | Small umbilicated vesicles/erosions | Face spared Burrows on fingers/wrists | Face involved

Exudate +++ | Extremely painful | Intensely itchy | Macules/papules/vesicles/pustules

ACUTE ECZEMA | ECZEMA HERPETICUM | SCABIES | CHICKEN POX

[p. 81] | [p. 81] | [p. 81] | [see p. 79]

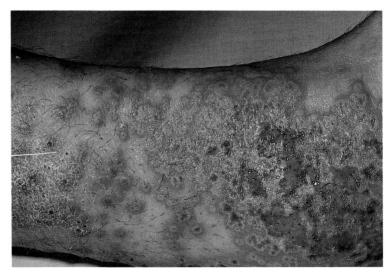

**4.10** Eczema herpeticum on the leg: umbilicated vesicles rupturing to leave circular painful erosions.

## ECZEMA HERPETICUM

Eczema may become secondarily infected with herpes simplex. The characteristic feature is small umbilicated vesicles which are painful rather than itchy. The patient will be more ill than might be expected from normal eczema. Swabs from the vesicles will confirm the presence of the herpes simplex virus.

## ACUTE ECZEMA

Acute eczema clinically presents with superficial vesicles which rapidly burst to produce exudate and crusts. It may be due to an acute flare of chronic atopic eczema (see p. 103), secondary infection of chronic eczema or a contact allergic eczema (see p. 45).

## SCABIES

Since scabies is extremely itchy, the rash on the trunk may become excoriated and crusted, and so be confused with a crusted eczema. It is important therefore to check the fingers for burrows (see p. 116).

**Trunk, limbs, face**
**Acute erythematous rash/lesions**
**Generalized rash (> 50% body involved)**
**1 Maculo-papular rashes (see p. 74)**
**2 Confluent widespread erythema**

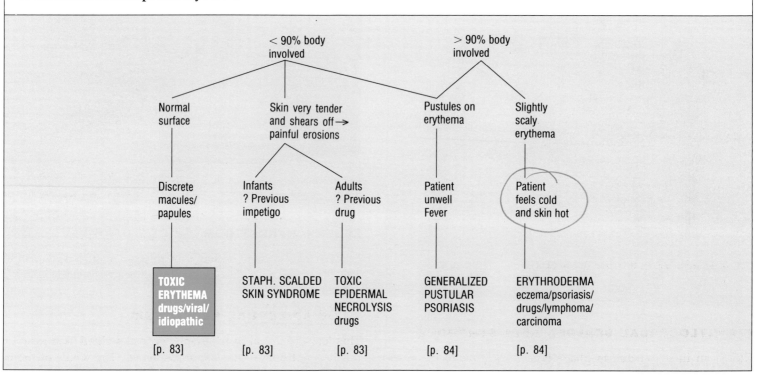

## TOXIC ERYTHEMA

Widespread maculo-papular rashes may be due to infection or drugs (see p. 74). Often the cause cannot be identified.

(see p. 74)

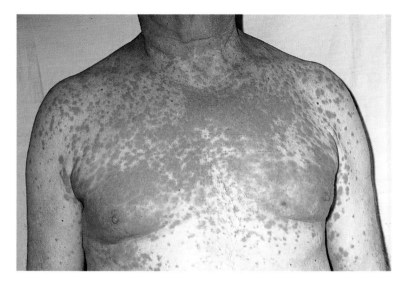

**4.12** Staphylococcal scalded skin syndrome.

**4.11** Toxic erythema, in this case due to Septrin.

## STAPHYLOCOCCAL SCALDED SKIN SYNDROME

This is an infection due to phage type 71 *Staphylococcus aureus* which produces a toxin which causes a split in the upper part of the epidermis. It occurs almost entirely in infants and young children. The skin becomes red and very tender (like a scald) and then peels off. It often begins in the flexures but usually spreads to involve the whole body.

## TOXIC EPIDERMAL NECROLYSIS

This looks identical to the staphylococcal scalded skin syndrome but it is not due to *Staphylococcus aureus*. The whole of the epidermis dies, leaving what appears to be a subepidermal blister. It occurs in adults and may be due to drugs such as the non-steroidal anti-inflammatory agents and sulphonamides, a lymphoma or be of unknown cause. It is much more serious than its childhood look-alike with a mortality of about 20 percent. Death occurs due to fluid loss or septicaemia. If large areas of the epidermis are lost, the patient will need to be treated like someone with an extensive burn, preferably in a burns unit.

## GENERALIZED PUSTULAR PSORIASIS

This acute, serious and unstable form of psoriasis is often precipitated by withdrawal of systemic or very potent topical steroids. Sheets of erythema studded with tiny sterile pustules come in waves associated with fever and general malaise. Such patients should be managed in hospital since there is a considerable mortality. This is the main reason psoriasis should not be treated with either topical or systemic steroids.

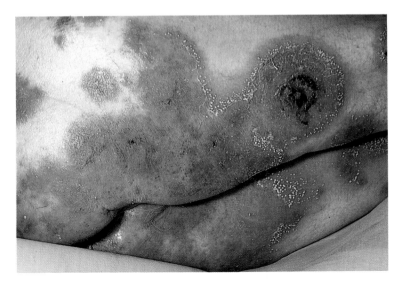

**4.13** Generalized pustular psoriasis.

## ERYTHRODERMA (EXFOLIATIVE DERMATITIS)

Erythroderma is the term used when the whole body is red and scaly. It may be due to eczema, psoriasis, a drug reaction, a carcinoma or a lymphoma. These patients too should be managed in hospital both to find the cause and prevent hypothermia.

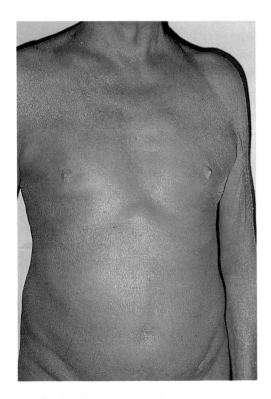

**4.14** Erythroderma: in this patient due to carcinoma of pancreas.

**Trunk and limbs**
**Chronic erythematous rash/lesions**
**Normal/smooth surface**
**Macules and patches**

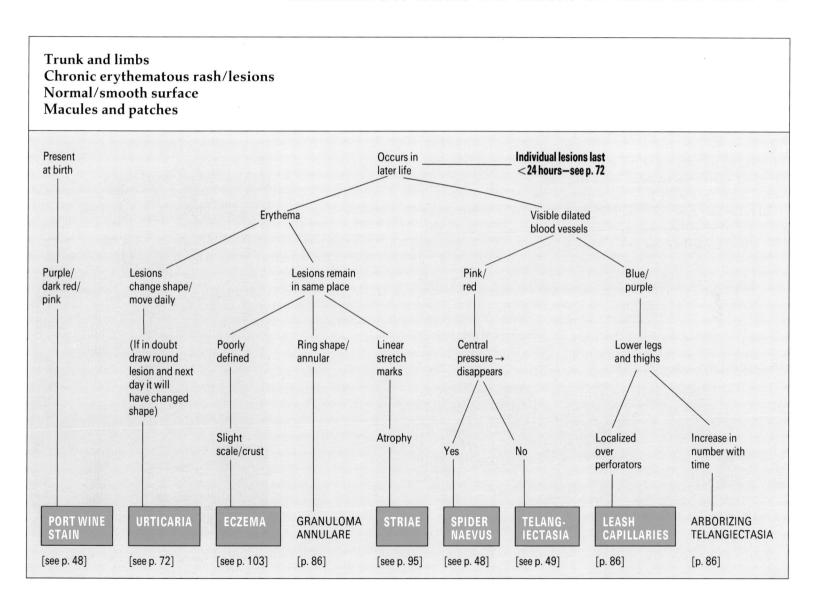

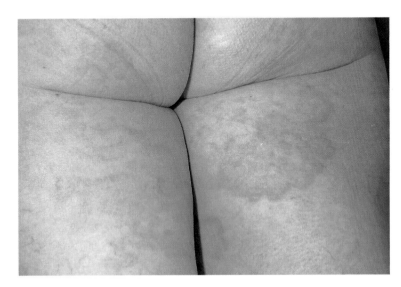

**4.15** Granuloma annulare: flat variety looking like a capillary haemangioma.

### GRANULOMA ANNULARE

Granuloma annulare occasionally presents as a flat area of discolouration on the skin. The colour ranges from pink to mauve. The surface is never scaly and there may be more typical papular lesions on the dorsum of the hands and feet (see p. 217). They remain static for many months or years but will eventually clear spontaneously.

### LEASH CAPILLARIES

Small areas of dilated veins on the lower legs are very common, especially in women over the age of 30 who have had children. They are unsightly but otherwise harmless.

### ARBORIZING TELANGIECTASIA

This is a progressive symmetrical dilatation of venules on the lower legs, gradually spreading upwards. The vessels form branches like a tree.

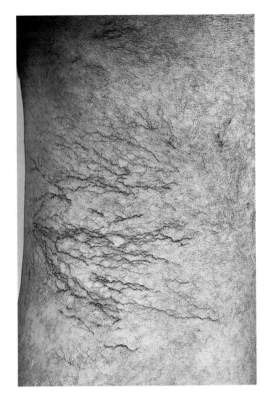

**4.16** Arborizing telangiectasia on lower leg.

**Trunk, limbs and face**
**Chronic erythematous lesions**
**Surface normal/smooth**
**1a Single or few (1–5) small papules (< 0.5 cm size)—No pustules**

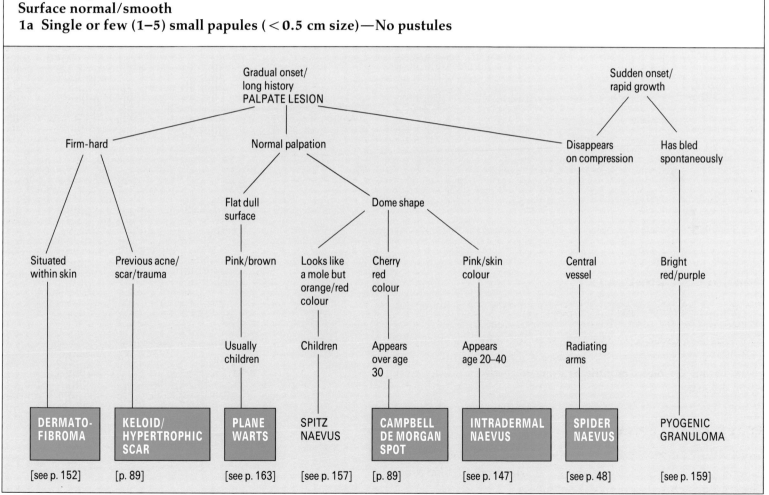

Gradual onset/
long history
PALPATE LESION

Sudden onset/
rapid growth

Firm-hard

Normal palpation

Disappears
on compression

Has bled
spontaneously

Flat dull
surface

Dome shape

Situated
within skin

Previous acne/
scar/trauma

Pink/brown

Looks like
a mole but
orange/red
colour

Cherry
red
colour

Pink/skin
colour

Central
vessel

Bright
red/purple

Usually
children

Children

Appears
over age
30

Appears
age 20–40

Radiating
arms

**DERMATO-FIBROMA**

**KELOID/HYPERTROPHIC SCAR**

**PLANE WARTS**

SPITZ
NAEVUS

**CAMPBELL DE MORGAN SPOT**

**INTRADERMAL NAEVUS**

**SPIDER NAEVUS**

PYOGENIC
GRANULOMA

[see p. 152]    [p. 89]    [see p. 163]    [see p. 157]    [p. 89]    [see p. 147]    [see p. 48]    [see p. 159]

**Trunk, limbs, face**
**Chronic erythematous rash/lesions**
**Surface normal**
**1b Single or few (1–5) large papules (>0.5cm size)/plaques/nodules—No pustules**

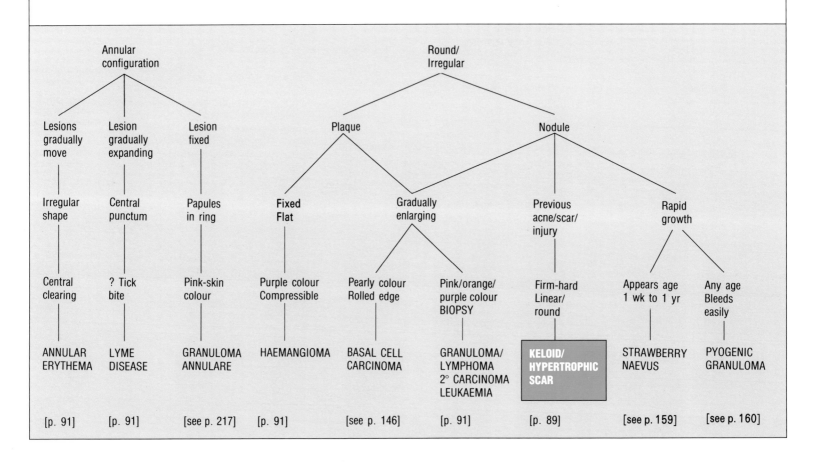

## CAMPBELL DE MORGAN SPOT (CHERRY ANGIOMA)

These small (1−4mm) bright red or purple papules appear on the trunk and proximal limbs after the age of 35. They are harmless.

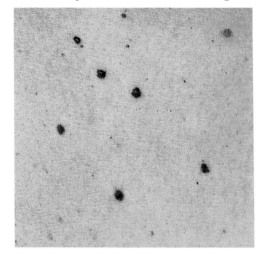

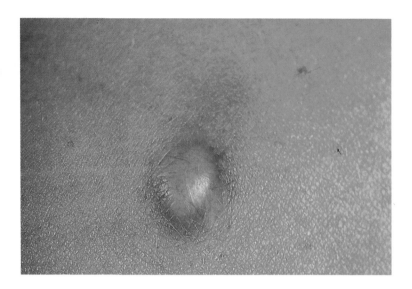

**4.17** Campbell de Morgan spots (cherry angiomas) on front of chest.

## KELOID AND HYPERTROPHIC SCARS

Hypertrophic scars are an overgrowth of scar tissue confined to the site of injury, while keloid scars grow out beyond the original site of injury. The commonest sites are on the front of chest and over the shoulders.

*Right above*
**4.18** Hypertrophic scar following BCG vaccination.

*Right below*
**4.19** Keloid scar following herpes zoster.

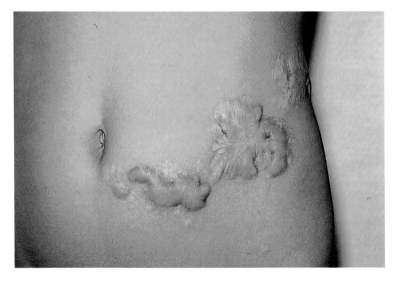

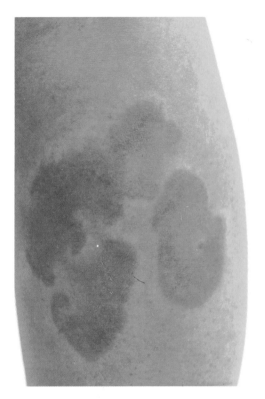

**4.20** Annular erythema, cause unknown.

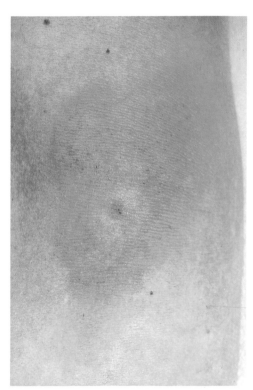

**4.21** Erythema chronicum migrans (Lyme disease): annular lesion with no scaling and an obvious bite in the centre.

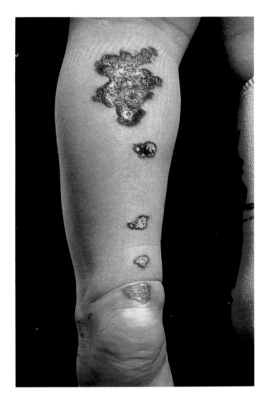

**4.22** Angiokeratoma on the left lower leg. It differs from an ordinary haemangioma in having a scaly surface.

## ANNULAR ERYTHEMA

This describes areas of erythema which are annular or figurate in shape. Over a period of days the areas of erythema gradually expand or change. The lesions are often scaly just inside the spreading edge.

## LYME DISEASE

A single lesion of gradually expanding annular erythema (erythema chronicum migrans) with a central punctum is likely to be Lyme disease. It is due to a tick bite which transmits a spirochaete (*Borrelia burgdorferi*) into the skin.

## HAEMANGIOMA

Vascular malformations may present as fixed plaques or nodules which are red or purple in colour. Firm compression of the lesion results in its partial emptying. Some lesions may be hyperkeratotic.

## GRANULOMATOUS, LYMPHOMATOUS, CARCINOMATOUS OR LEUKAEMIC INFILTRATES

Any indurated erythematous papule or nodule that remains fixed for a period of time should be biopsied. This will distinguish the benign infiltrates from malignant lesions.

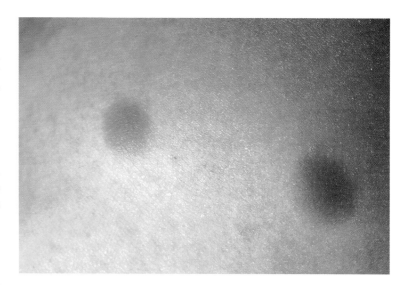

*Right above*
**4.23** Leukaemic infiltrate in the skin (acute monoblastic leukaemia): diagnosis made by skin biopsy.

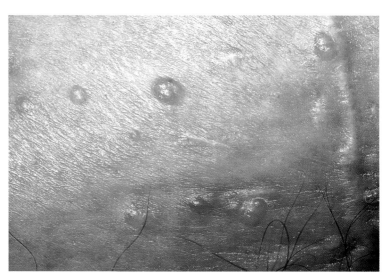

*Right below*
**4.24** Papules on the abdominal wall due to secondary carcinoma. Note nearby scar from original operation (carcinoma of ovary).

**Trunks and limbs**
**Chronic erythematous rash/lesions**
**Surface normal/smooth**
**2a  Widespread/multiple small papules (< 0.5 cm size)—No pustules**

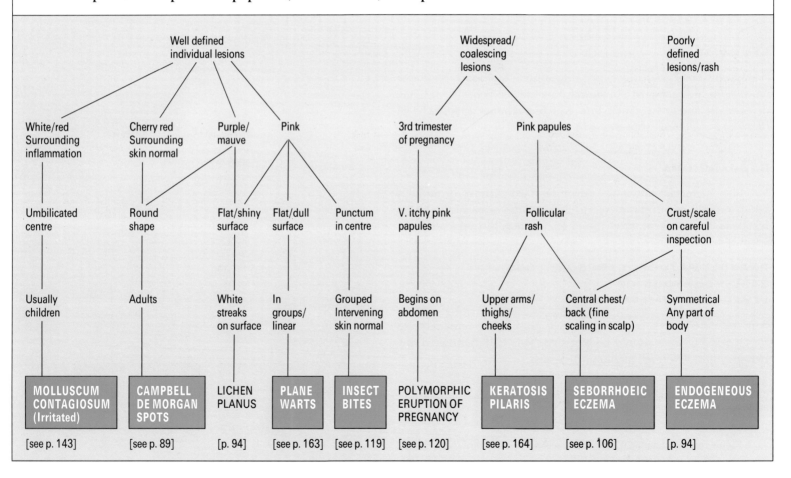

**Trunk and limbs**
**Chronic erythematous rash/lesions**
**Surface normal/smooth**
**2b  Widespread/multiple large papules (> 0.5 cm size)/plaques/nodules—No pustules**

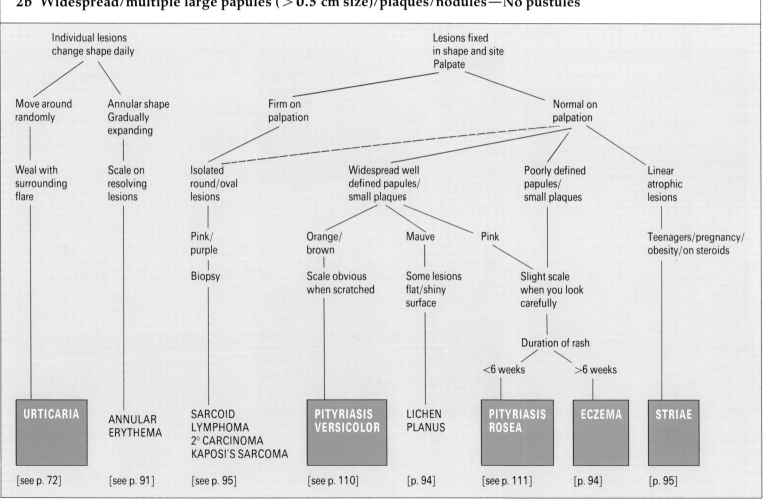

Individual lesions
change shape daily

Lesions fixed
in shape and site
Palpate

Move around
randomly

Annular shape
Gradually
expanding

Firm on
palpation

Normal on
palpation

Weal with
surrounding
flare

Scale on
resolving
lesions

Isolated
round/oval
lesions

Widespread well
defined papules/
small plaques

Poorly defined
papules/
small plaques

Linear
atrophic
lesions

Pink/
purple

Orange/
brown

Mauve

Pink

Teenagers/pregnancy/
obesity/on steroids

Biopsy

Scale obvious
when scratched

Some lesions
flat/shiny
surface

Slight scale
when you look
carefully

Duration of rash

<6 weeks    >6 weeks

**URTICARIA**

ANNULAR
ERYTHEMA

SARCOID
LYMPHOMA
2° CARCINOMA
KAPOSI'S SARCOMA

**PITYRIASIS
VERSICOLOR**

LICHEN
PLANUS

**PITYRIASIS
ROSEA**

**ECZEMA**

**STRIAE**

[see p. 72]    [see p. 91]    [see p. 95]    [see p. 110]    [p. 94]    [see p. 111]    [p. 94]    [p. 95]

## ECZEMA

The scaling in eczema may not be obvious but is usually there if carefully looked for (see p. 103).

## LICHEN PLANUS

Lesions in lichen planus are small mauve, flat-topped, shiny papules which sometimes have white streaky areas on the surface

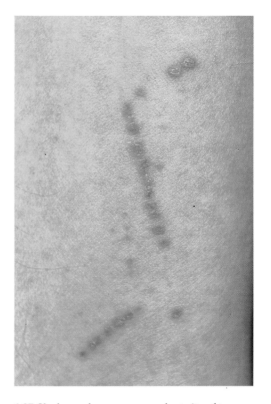

**4.25** Lichen planus: typical flat topped shiny papules.

**4.26** Lichen planus on back of hand showing white lace-like pattern on surface (Wickham's striae).

**4.27** Koebner phenomenon: rash at site of trauma. Occurs with lichen planus, psoriasis and plane warts.

(Wickham's striae). The most characteristic place to look for the rash is on the flexor aspect of the wrist, but it is usually widespread on the trunk and limbs, and may occur at sites of trauma such as scratch marks or operation scars (Koebner phenomenon). Although it is very itchy, excoriations are not usually seen. As the rash gets better the colour of the papules changes from mauve to brown. The buccal mucosa and tongue may be involved with a white lace-like streaky pattern which will not scrape off with a spatula. The rash can last 9–18 months before disappearing. There may be some residual post-inflammatory hyperpigmentation.

## STRIAE

Linear red/purple plaques occur commonly on the thighs and lumbosacral region in teenagers. With time they flatten off and become atrophic. Similar lesions occur on the abdomen and breasts in pregnancy, and in the flexures in patients on systemic steroids or using potent topical steroids.

## SARCOID/LYMPHOMA/SECONDARY CARCINOMA

Multiple papules on the trunk and limbs may be due to sarcoid. If you suspect this, X-ray the chest and do a skin biopsy.

Lymphoma and secondary deposits of a carcinoma may present on the skin as non-compressible skin-coloured or purplish papules, plaques and nodules: the diagnosis is made by a skin biopsy.

Kaposi's sarcoma: see p. 160.

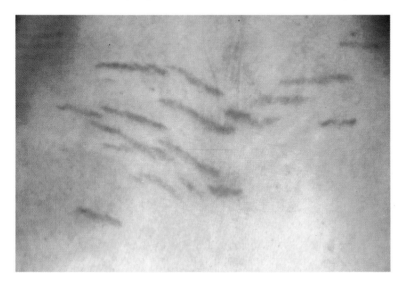

**4.28** Adolescent striae on lower back in a 17 year old boy.

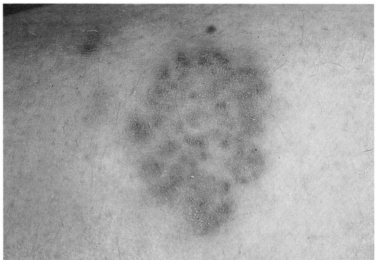

**4.29** Sarcoid papules on the leg: mauve colour with no surface scale. Confirm diagnosis by biopsy.

**Trunk and limbs
Chronic erythematous rash/lesions
Surface normal
Papules, nodules and pustules**

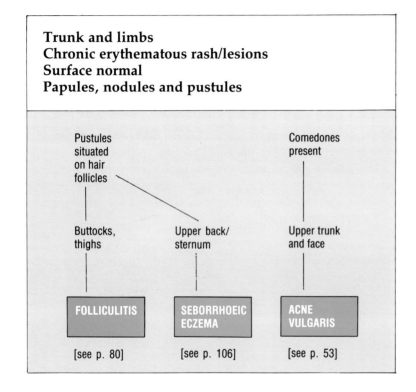

Pustules situated on hair follicles

Comedones present

Buttocks, thighs

Upper back/ sternum

Upper trunk and face

| FOLLICULITIS | SEBORRHOEIC ECZEMA | ACNE VULGARIS |
|---|---|---|

[see p. 80]    [see p. 106]    [see p. 53]

**Trunk and limbs
Chronic erythematous rash/lesions
Scaly surface
Papules and plaques**

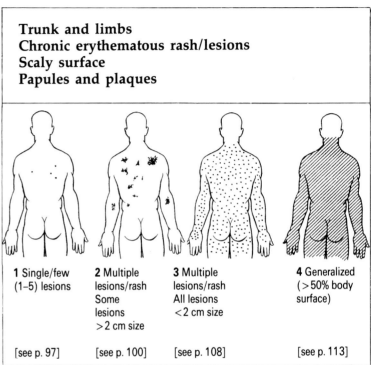

**1** Single/few (1–5) lesions

**2** Multiple lesions/rash Some lesions >2 cm size

**3** Multiple lesions/rash All lesions <2 cm size

**4** Generalized (>50% body surface)

[see p. 97]    [see p. 100]    [see p. 108]    [see p. 113]

**Trunk and limbs**
**Chronic erythematous lesions**
**Scaly surface**
**1 Single/few (1–5) papules & plaques (nodules see p. 167)**

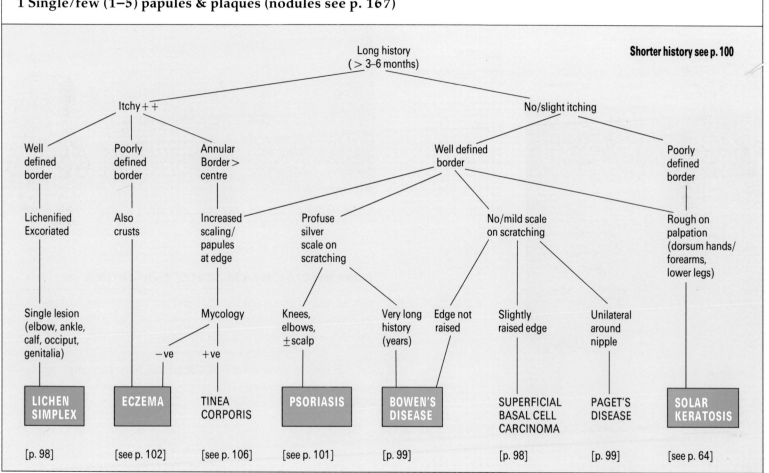

Long history
( > 3–6 months)

**Shorter history see p. 100**

Itchy + +

No/slight itching

Well defined border

Poorly defined border

Annular Border > centre

Well defined border

Poorly defined border

Lichenified Excoriated

Also crusts

Increased scaling/ papules at edge

Profuse silver scale on scratching

No/mild scale on scratching

Rough on palpation (dorsum hands/ forearms, lower legs)

Single lesion (elbow, ankle, calf, occiput, genitalia)

Mycology

Knees, elbows, ±scalp

Very long history (years)

Edge not raised

Slightly raised edge

Unilateral around nipple

−ve       +ve

| LICHEN SIMPLEX | ECZEMA | TINEA CORPORIS | PSORIASIS | BOWEN'S DISEASE | | SUPERFICIAL BASAL CELL CARCINOMA | PAGET'S DISEASE | SOLAR KERATOSIS |

[p. 98]   [see p. 102]   [see p. 106]   [see p. 101]   [p. 99]   [p. 98]   [p. 99]   [see p. 64]

## LICHEN SIMPLEX

Lichen simplex is a single, well-defined itchy plaque with increased skin markings on the surface (lichenification) due to persistent scratching. If the patient stops scratching it will heal, but this is often easier said than done. The commonest sites are the occiput, ankles, elbows and genitalia.

**4.30** Lichen simplex on elbow: unilateral, increased skin markings and no silvery scaling differentiates this from psoriasis.

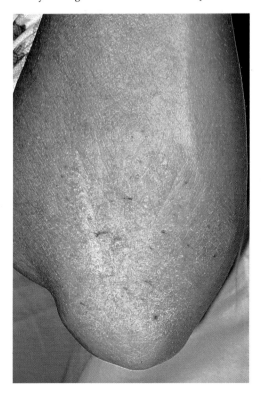

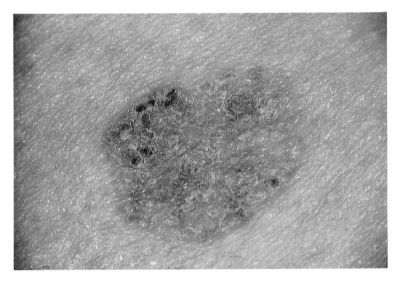

**4.31** Superficial basal cell carcinoma: note rolled translucent edge to lesion.

## SUPERFICIAL BASAL CELL CARCINOMA

On the trunk, basal cell carcinomas (BCCS) often spread superficially and slowly over several years, presenting as a flat scaly plaque. The edge of the lesion is just like a BCC elsewhere with a slightly raised, rolled edge; this can be seen more easily if the skin is put on the stretch. The centre of the lesion may be scaly and can be confused with Bowen's disease, or even eczema. A biopsy will distinguish between them.

## BOWEN'S DISEASE

This is an intra-epidermal squamous cell carcinoma. It looks just like a plaque of psoriasis or eczema, but gradually expands in size over many years and does not respond to topical steroids. The lower leg is the commonest site, but it can be found anywhere on the skin surface.

If multiple lesions are present, particularly if they are not on sun-exposed sites, arsenic rather than ultra-violet light may be the cause. Previous arsenic ingestion is confirmed by the presence of rough warty papules on the palms and soles (arsenical keratoses).

## PAGET'S DISEASE OF THE NIPPLE

This is due to invasion of the skin around the nipple by malignant cells derived from an intraduct carcinoma. There is a unilateral red scaly plaque surrounding the nipple with or without crusting. It gradually increases in size and is often mistaken for eczema. The fact that is it unilateral and does not respond to topical steroids should alert you to the diagnosis.

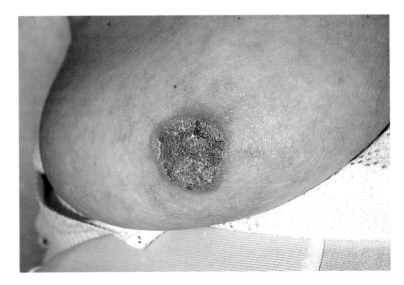

**4.33** Paget's disease of the nipple (courtesy of Dr. P Goodwin.)

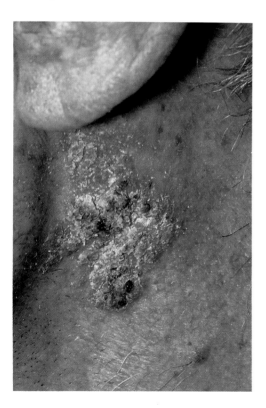

**4.32** Bowen's disease.

**Trunk and limbs**
**Chronic erythematous rash/lesions**
**Scaly surface**
**Papules and plaques (nodules see p. 167)**
**2  Multiple lesions/rash—Some lesions > 2 cm size (all lesions < 2 cm size see p.108)**

Scratch rash vigorously with nail; note colour

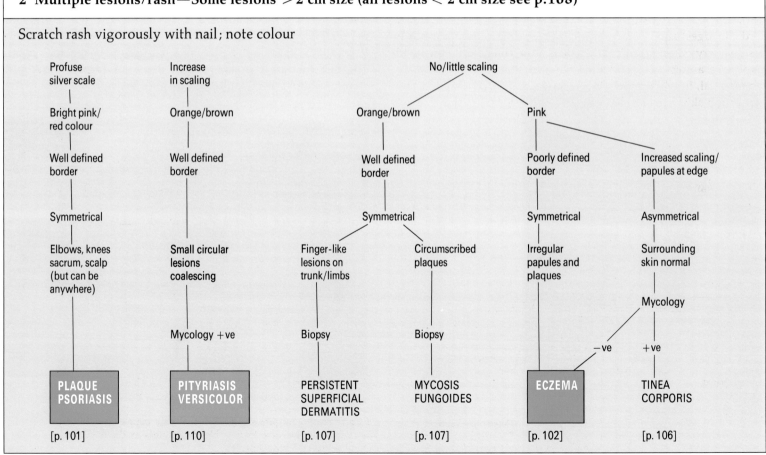

| | | | | | |
|---|---|---|---|---|---|
| Profuse silver scale | Increase in scaling | | No/little scaling | | |
| Bright pink/red colour | Orange/brown | Orange/brown | | Pink | |
| Well defined border | Well defined border | Well defined border | | Poorly defined border | Increased scaling/papules at edge |
| Symmetrical | | Symmetrical | | Symmetrical | Asymmetrical |
| Elbows, knees sacrum, scalp (but can be anywhere) | Small circular lesions coalescing | Finger-like lesions on trunk/limbs | Circumscribed plaques | Irregular papules and plaques | Surrounding skin normal |
| | | | | | Mycology |
| | Mycology +ve | Biopsy | Biopsy | —ve | +ve |
| **PLAQUE PSORIASIS** | **PITYRIASIS VERSICOLOR** | PERSISTENT SUPERFICIAL DERMATITIS | MYCOSIS FUNGOIDES | **ECZEMA** | TINEA CORPORIS |
| [p. 101] | [p. 110] | [p. 107] | [p. 107] | [p. 102] | [p. 106] |

## CHRONIC PLAQUE PSORIASIS

Psoriasis is a common disease which affects about 2 percent of the population worldwide. It can occur at any age but most often begins between the ages of 15 and 25 years.

The clinical features can be explained by the pathology (Fig. 4.34). The lesions are bright red in colour, have clearly defined borders (edges) and a silvery scale. The scale becomes more obviously silvery when scratched, and the scale comes off easily and may make a mess on the floor. Characteristically the lesions are symmetrical, involving the elbows, knees and sacral area, but any part of the skin can be involved including the scalp and nails.

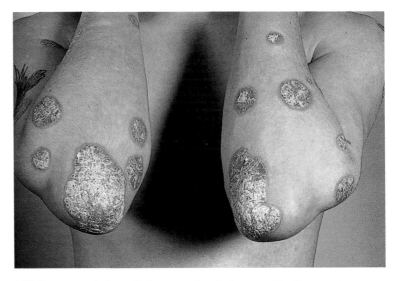

**4.35** Plaque psoriasis: well demarcated red plaques with silvery scale.

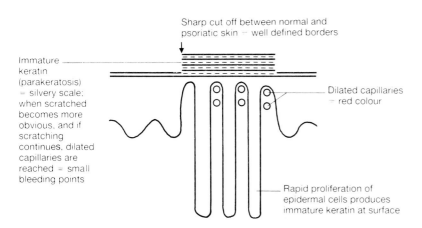

**4.34** Pathology of psoriasis.

Sharp cut off between normal and psoriatic skin = well defined borders

Immature keratin (parakeratosis) = silvery scale; when scratched becomes more obvious, and if scratching continues, dilated capillaries are reached = small bleeding points

Dilated capillaries = red colour

Rapid proliferation of epidermal cells produces immature keratin at surface

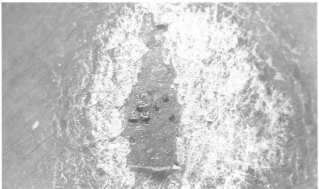

**4.36** Psoriasis: Auspitz sign. When the scaly plaque is scratched, you very quickly come to tiny bleeding points as the few layers of epidermal cells are removed.

# Chronic eczema

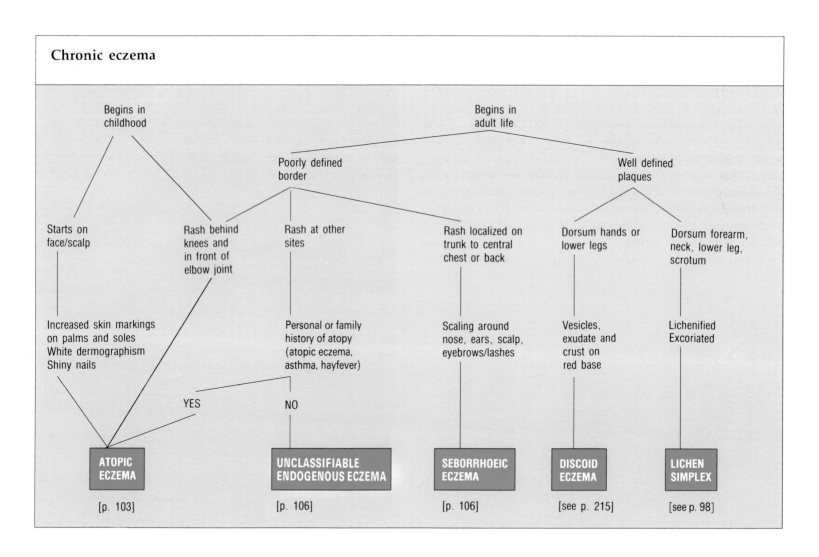

Begins in childhood

Begins in adult life

Poorly defined border

Well defined plaques

Starts on face/scalp

Rash behind knees and in front of elbow joint

Rash at other sites

Rash localized on trunk to central chest or back

Dorsum hands or lower legs

Dorsum forearm, neck, lower leg, scrotum

Increased skin markings on palms and soles
White dermographism
Shiny nails

Personal or family history of atopy (atopic eczema, asthma, hayfever)

Scaling around nose, ears, scalp, eyebrows/lashes

Vesicles, exudate and crust on red base

Lichenified
Excoriated

YES

NO

**ATOPIC ECZEMA**

**UNCLASSIFIABLE ENDOGENOUS ECZEMA**

**SEBORRHOEIC ECZEMA**

**DISCOID ECZEMA**

**LICHEN SIMPLEX**

[p. 103]

[p. 106]

[p. 106]

[see p. 215]

[see p. 98]

## CHRONIC ECZEMA

In this book the term eczema is used for both the endogenous eczemas, and those due to external factors since the word dermatitis has industrial and litigation connotations. The word eczema comes from the Greek word meaning 'to bubble through', and the hallmark of eczema is the presence of vesicles. In practice vesicles are only seen in acute eczema (Fig. 4.37), but the patient will often tell you that small blisters have been present in the past. What you normally see is a poorly defined pink scaly rash which is very itchy. It is distinguished from psoriasis by being much less vivid in colour (usually a nondescript pink), with poorly defined edges and less obvious scale. Scaling will be present but does not become either more obvious or silvery in colour when scratched.

## ATOPIC ECZEMA

Atopy means an inherited predisposition to eczema, asthma or hayfever, and atopic individuals may have one or all of these manifestations.

The eczema usually begins between the ages of 3 and 12 months, the asthma at age 3–4 years and the hayfever in the teens. In infancy the eczema often begins on the scalp and face, and may or may not spread to involve the rest of the body. When children get

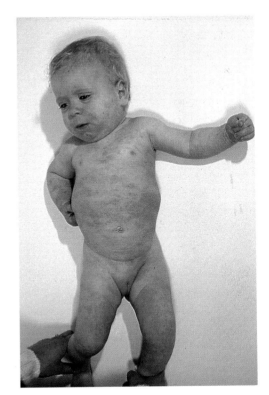

4.38 Atopic eczema: widespread rash in a 9-month-old girl.

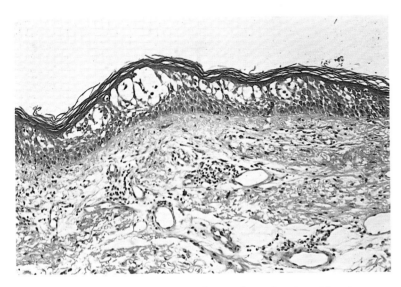

4.37 Pathology of acute eczema: note the vesicles within the epidermis.

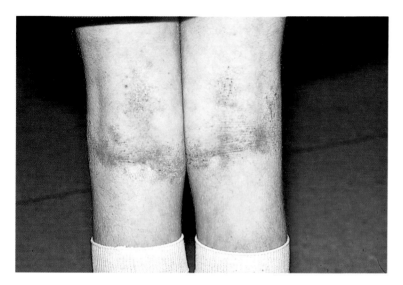

**4.39** Atopic eczema: localized to flexures in a 7-year-old girl.

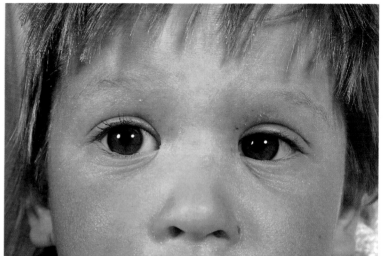

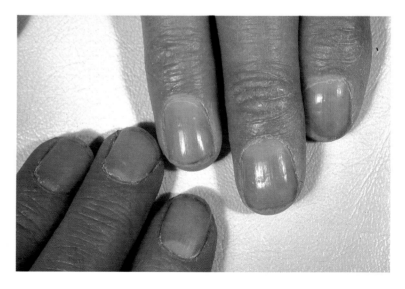

older it may localize in the flexures, particularly the popliteal and antecubital fossae. It is very itchy so excoriations and lichenification may be seen, and if the children rub rather than scratch, the nails may be very shiny. Fifty percent of such children will also have ichthyosis (dry scaly skin) and increased skin markings on the palms and soles.

In 90 percent of children the eczema will clear spontaneously by puberty, but in a small minority, it will persist into adult life. A few of these will have very extensive and troublesome eczema all

*Right above*
**4.40** Atopic eczema: poorly defined pink scaly rash. Note the increased skin crease under the eyes which is typical of atopic eczema in children.

*Right below*
**4.41** Atopic eczema shiny nails due to continual rubbing (top fingers).

their lives. For others there is a period during the teens when the skin is clear, only for it to return in the 20s. The causes for worsening of atopic eczema are given in Table 4.1.

In adults a diagnosis of atopic eczema can be made if there is a history of infantile eczema, or if they also have or have had asthma, hayfever, ichthyosis, increased skin markings on their palms and soles or white dermographism (stroke gently with your finger nail through an area of eczema: after 30 seconds a white line appears). A positive history of atopic eczema or asthma in the immediate family (parents, siblings, children) is further evidence of atopy.

**Table 4.1.** Causes of worsening of atopic eczema.

1 Cold weather
2 Treatment not used regularly
3 Emotional upset
4 Secondary infection with bacteria or herpes simplex virus
5 Patient has scabies or some other itchy rash too.

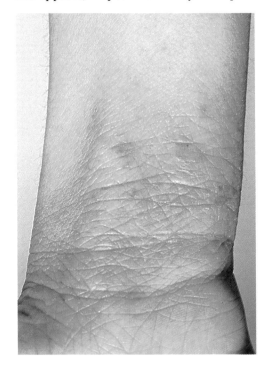

**4.42** Atopic eczema: lichenification at wrist due to continual scratching.

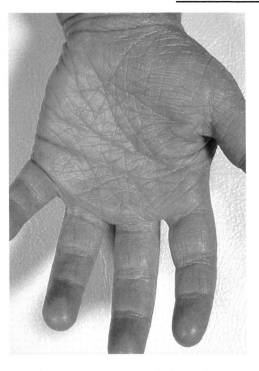

**4.43** Atopic eczema: increased skin markings on palm.

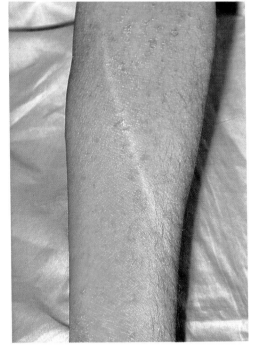

**4.44** Atopic eczema: white dermographism.

## SEBORRHOEIC ECZEMA

The diagnosis of seborrhoeic eczema is made on the distribution of the rash. The scalp is always involved with scaling and/or redness. The eyebrows, eyelashes, external ears and naso-labial folds are often also involved. On the trunk pink or orangey-brown poorly defined scaly plaques are present on the centre of the chest or back, and occasionally in the flexures (see pp. 65, 175). Less commonly, small follicular papules are the predominant feature on the trunk.

## UNCLASSIFIABLE ECZEMA

Eczema on the trunk and limbs which does not fit one of the patterns described above is called unclassifiable endogenous eczema.

## TINEA CORPORIS (RINGWORM)

Ringworm of the body is due to dermatophyte fungi of the *Microsporum*, *Trichophyton* and *Epidermophyton* species. Dermatophytes live on keratin and cause a pink scaly plaque. The lesion tends to spread outwards as the stratum corneum is used up leaving less scaly skin in the middle, hence the name ringworm. It does not always form a ring, and the diagnosis of tinea should be considered in any *asymmetrical* red scaly rash.

If the lesion is viewed from a distance of about 6 feet, there is a definite border consisting of increased scaling or papules: outside this the skin is normal. Treatment with steroids will alter the clinical appearance making the centre of the ring more uniform and less scaly (tinea incognito).

The diagnosis of tinea can be confirmed by examination of skin scales from the edge of the lesion (see p. 9).

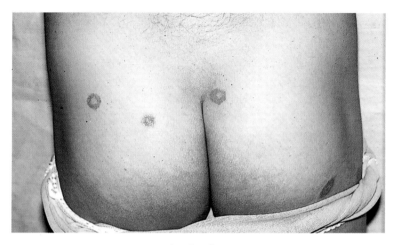

4.45 Tinea corporis: asymmetrical red scaly rings.

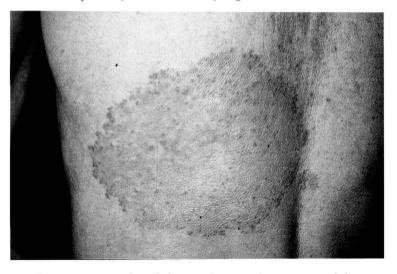

4.46 Tinea incognito: unilateral plaque with active edge, some central clearing. Lack of scaling due to application of topical steroids.

## MYCOSIS FUNGOIDES

This uncommon disease is a T-cell lymphoma confined to the skin. It presents as red scaly plaques that may mimic either eczema or psoriasis. The main differentiating feature is that individual lesions are of different colours, so that some plaques are pink, others red or orangey brown. This stage of mycosis fungoides may persist for many years, but eventually tumours develop from the plaques and the disease may then spread to other organs of the body. The diagnosis is confirmed by skin biopsy.

## PERSISTENT SUPERFICIAL DERMATITIS

This is similar to the early stages of mycosis fungoides with persistent oblong or finger-shaped plaques around the trunk. It differs from mycosis fungoides in that the lesions are all the same colour and a biopsy will show eczema and not lymphoma.

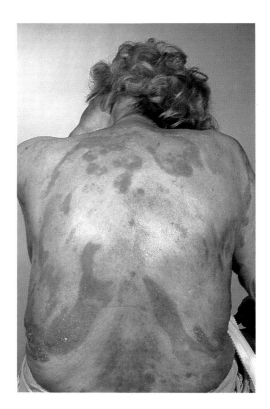

4.47 Mycosis fungoides: plaques of differing colours.

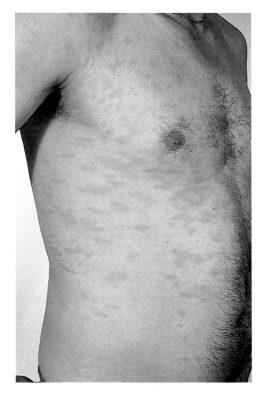

4.48 Persistent superficial dermatitis: fixed finger shaped plaques around trunk.

**Trunk and limbs**
**Chronic erythematous lesions/rash**
**Scaly surface**
**Papules and plaques (< 2 cm)**
**3 Multiple lesions/rash—all lesions less than 2 cm size**

Scratch lesions firmly with nail, note colour and palpate with finger tips

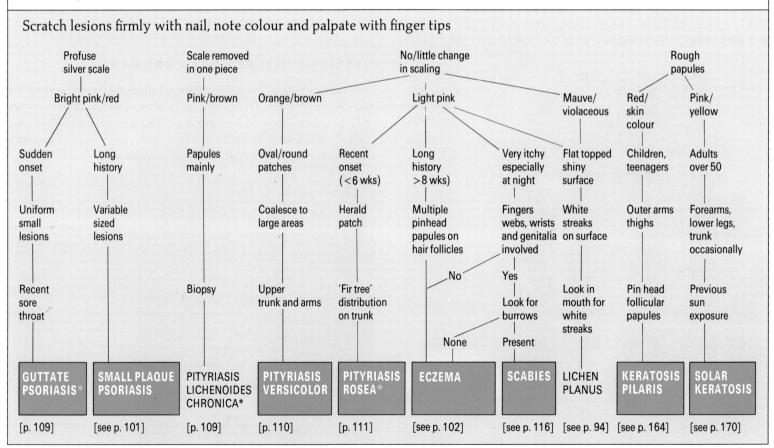

| | | | | | | | | | | |
|---|---|---|---|---|---|---|---|---|---|---|
| Profuse silver scale | | Scale removed in one piece | | | No/little change in scaling | | | | Rough papules | |
| Bright pink/red | | Pink/brown | Orange/brown | | Light pink | | | Mauve/ violaceous | Red/ skin colour | Pink/ yellow |
| Sudden onset | Long history | Papules mainly | Oval/round patches | Recent onset (<6 wks) | Long history >8 wks) | Very itchy especially at night | Flat topped shiny surface | Children, teenagers | Adults over 50 |
| Uniform small lesions | Variable sized lesions | | Coalesce to large areas | Herald patch | Multiple pinhead papules on hair follicles | Fingers webs, wrists and genitalia involved | White streaks on surface | Outer arms thighs | Forearms, lower legs, trunk occasionally |
| | | | | | | No / Yes | | | |
| Recent sore throat | | Biopsy | Upper trunk and arms | 'Fir tree' distribution on trunk | | Look for burrows | Look in mouth for white streaks | Pin head follicular papules | Previous sun exposure |
| | | | | | | None / Present | | | |
| **GUTTATE PSORIASIS***  | **SMALL PLAQUE PSORIASIS** | PITYRIASIS LICHENOIDES CHRONICA* | **PITYRIASIS VERSICOLOR** | **PITYRIASIS ROSEA***  | **ECZEMA** | **SCABIES** | LICHEN PLANUS | **KERATOSIS PILARIS** | **SOLAR KERATOSIS** |
| [p. 109] | [see p. 101] | [p. 109] | [p. 110] | [p. 111] | [see p. 102] | [see p. 116] | [see p. 94] | [see p. 164] | [see p. 170] |

*If patient unwell, has palmar lesions and lymphadenopathy consider SECONDARY SYPHILIS (p. 112).

## GUTTATE PSORIASIS

This is an acute form of psoriasis that appears suddenly 10—14 days after a streptococcal sore throat. The individual lesions are typical of psoriasis, being bright red, well demarcated with silvery scaling, but are uniformly small (0.5—1.0 cm in diameter). The rash may be very widespread, comes up more or less overnight and gets better spontaneously after 2—3 months. It may be the first manifestation of psoriasis or occur in someone who has had psoriasis for years.

Since it is usually not itchy, it can be confused with pityriasis rosea and secondary syphilis. Pityriasis rosea is a lighter pink colour and the scaling is around the edge of the plaques. Patients with secondary syphilis are unwell, have lymphadenopathy and often lesions on the palms and soles.

## PITYRIASIS LICHENOIDES CHRONICA

This rash is probably quite common but is rarely recognized by non-dermatologists. It consists of widespread small red-brown scaly papules, from which the scale can be 'picked off' in one piece. It is more common in children and young adults and lasts for several months; it often improves in the sun.

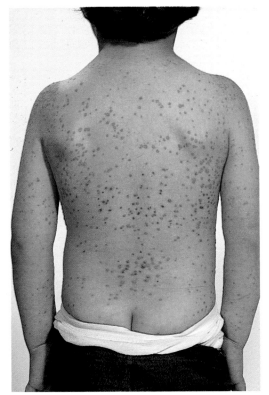

*Left*
**4.49** Guttate psoriasis: uniformly distributed small red scaly lesions.

*Right*
**4.50** Pityriasis lichenoides chronica: small red-brown scaly papules with scale that can be picked off in one piece.

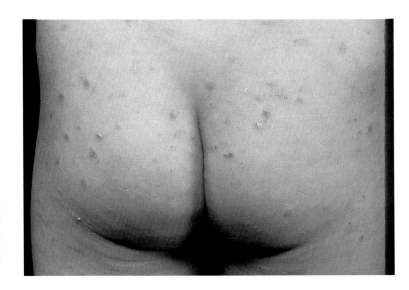

## PITYRIASIS VERSICOLOR

The word pityriasis means bran-like and is used for a scaly rash; versicolor means different colours. Pityriasis versicolor is therefore a scaly rash of different colours. In different individuals it may be white, orange-brown or dark brown. The lesions are small, less than 1 cm in diameter, usually round and always scaly when scratched. Some may join together to form larger confluent plaques. It is a disease of young adults and occurs predominantly on the upper trunk.

It is due to an infection with a yeast, *Pityrosporon orbiculare*, which we all have on our skin as a harmless commensal. Under certain conditions, the yeast produces hyphae and becomes pathogenic; it is then called *Malassezia furfur*. Most people with the rash have picked up the pathogenic form of the organism from someone else, possibly when on holiday in a warm climate. It is possible to transform your own commensal organisms if you are on steroids or other immunosuppressive therapy.

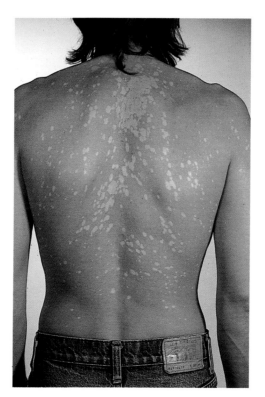

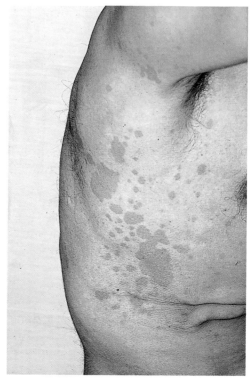

*Right*
**4.51** Pityriasis versicolor: white variety — hypopigmented areas.

*Far right*
**4.52** Pityriasis versicolor: orange-brown variety.

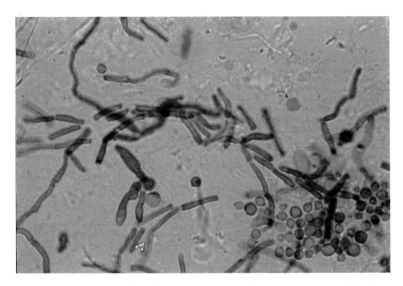

4.53 Pityriasis versicolor: direct microscopy showing spores and hyphae (Parker ink stain).

The orange-brown variety can be confused with pityriasis rosea but the diagnosis can be easily confirmed by scraping off the scales, mixing them with mixture of equal parts of 20 percent potassium hydroxide solution and Parker blue-black ink. The organism takes up the blue colour of the ink and both spores and hyphae are seen (Fig. 4.53). It is not possible to grow the organism on culture.

## PITYRIASIS ROSEA

This rash occurs in otherwise fit and healthy children or young adults, and lasts about 6 weeks. Firstly a single oval scaly plaque, usually 2–3 cm in diameter, appears on the trunk or on a limb (the herald patch); it may initially be misdiagnosed as ringworm.

A few days later, the rest of the rash appears. It consists of 2 different kinds of lesions:
1 Small pink follicular papules.
2 Petaloid lesions. These are similar to the herald patch but smaller: oval, pink, scaly macules or plaques where the scale is just inside the edge of the lesion.

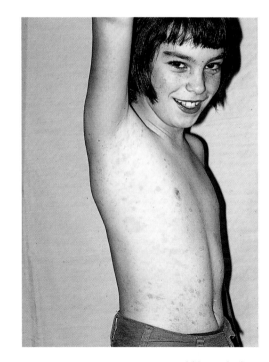

4.54 Pityriasis rosea in a 10-year-old boy: the herald patch is larger than the others. The rash follows the skin lines around the trunk.

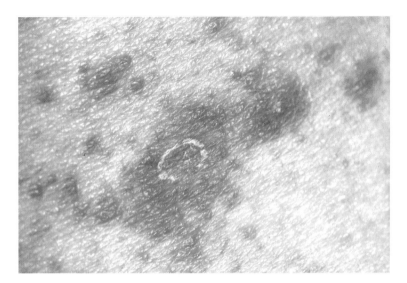

**4.55** Pityriasis rosea: two types of lesion.
1. Small follicular papules.
2. Early petaloid lesion with scale just beginning to move out towards the edge of the plaque.

If the herald patch is on the trunk, the rest of the rash is confined to the vest and pants area, and the individual lesions follow Langer's lines giving a 'Christmas tree' pattern. If the herald patch is on a limb, the rash may be mainly on the limbs; if the herald patch is on the neck, most of the rash may be on the face and trunk.

If the patient has a rash that looks like pitryiasis rosea but is unwell, think of secondary syphilis and check the VDRL.

## SECONDARY SYPHILIS

Secondary syphilis occurs about 6 weeks after a primary infection. The skin lesions are preceded by a flu-like illness and painless lymphadenopathy. The rash is very variable and may consist of macules, papules, pustules and plaques ranging in colour from pink to mauve, orange or brown. There are often lesions on the

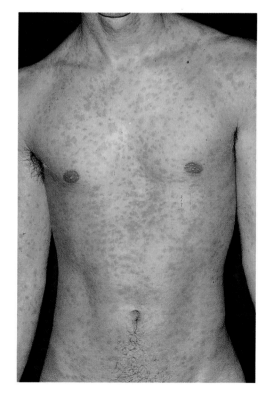

**4.56** Secondary syphilis on trunk.

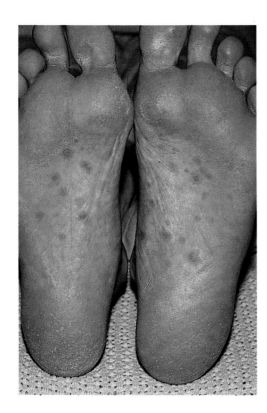

**4.57** Secondary syphilis on soles.

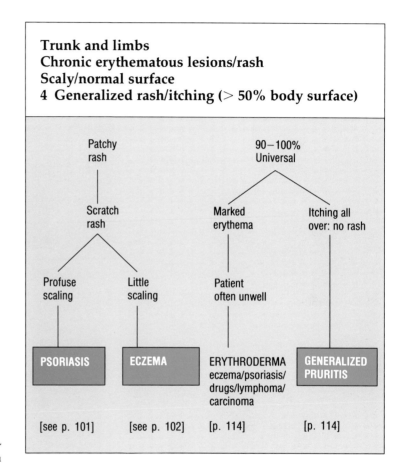

palms and soles. The diagnosis can be confirmed by a +ve VDRL which will distinguish it from all the other non-itchy rashes on the skin.

## ERYTHRODERMA

Total involvement of the body with a red scaly rash is termed erythroderma. This can occur suddenly or gradually over a period of months. The commonest causes are eczema, psoriasis and drug rashes. Rarely it may be due to an underlying lymphoma or carcinoma (see Fig. 4.14, p. 84).

## GENERALIZED PRURITIS

If someone is itching all over but no rash is seen other than excoriations consider:

1 Anaemia — especially iron deficiency
2 Uraemia
3 Obstructive jaundice
4 Thyroid disease — both hypo and hyperthyroidism
5 Lymphoma — especially in young adult (X-ray chest)
6 Carcinoma — especially in middle/old age
7 Body lice — look in seams of underwear for lice
8 Psychological.

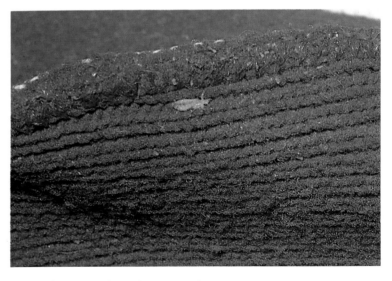

**4.58** Body louse and nits along seam of jumper.

**Trunk and limbs**
**Chronic erythematous lesions/rash**
**Excoriated surface or intense itching**
**Papules/plaques/nodules**

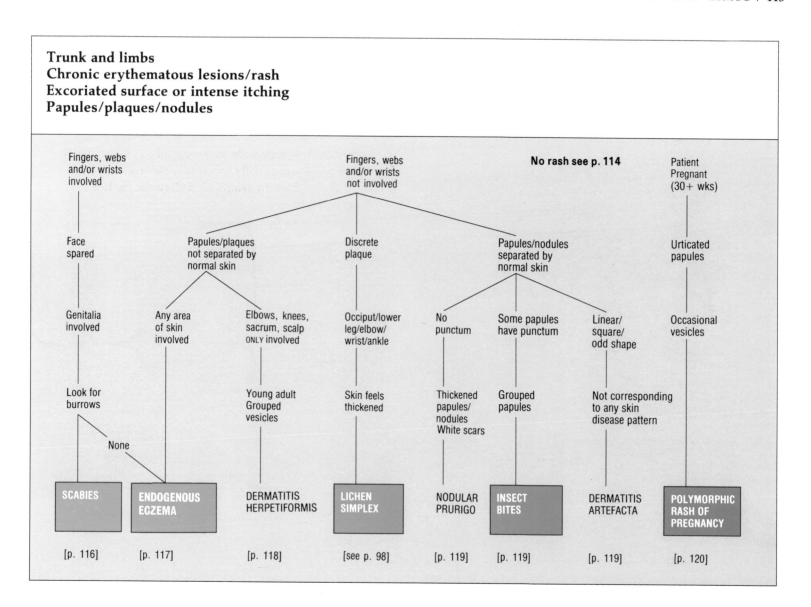

Fingers, webs and/or wrists involved

Face spared

Genitalia involved

Look for burrows

None

**SCABIES**

[p. 116]

Fingers, webs and/or wrists not involved

Papules/plaques not separated by normal skin

Any area of skin involved

**ENDOGENOUS ECZEMA**

[p. 117]

Elbows, knees, sacrum, scalp ONLY involved

Young adult Grouped vesicles

DERMATITIS HERPETIFORMIS

[p. 118]

Discrete plaque

Occiput/lower leg/elbow/wrist/ankle

Skin feels thickened

**LICHEN SIMPLEX**

[see p. 98]

No rash see p. 114

Papules/nodules separated by normal skin

No punctum

Thickened papules/nodules White scars

NODULAR PRURIGO

[p. 119]

Some papules have punctum

Grouped papules

**INSECT BITES**

[p. 119]

Linear/square/odd shape

Not corresponding to any skin disease pattern

DERMATITIS ARTEFACTA

[p. 119]

Patient Pregnant (30+ wks)

Urticated papules

Occasional vesicles

**POLYMORPHIC RASH OF PREGNANCY**

[p. 120]

## SCABIES

Scabies is an infestation with the human scabies mite, *Sarcoptes scabei* (Fig. 4.59). It is transmitted by prolonged contact with the skin of someone who is infested. A fertilized female (life cycle Fig. 4.60) has to be transferred for infection to take place. She will then find a place to lay her eggs (a burrow). Six to eight weeks later a secondary hypersensitivity rash occurs, characterized by intense itching particularly at night: this is usually made up of excoriated papules scattered over the trunk and limbs but sparing the face (except in infants).

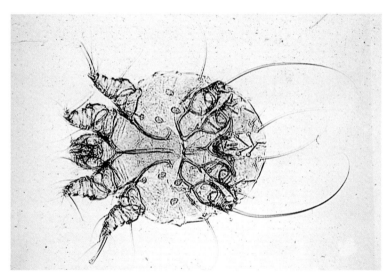

**4.59** Scabies mite (× 120).

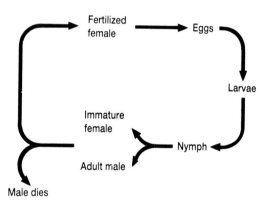

**4.60** Life cycle of scabies mite.

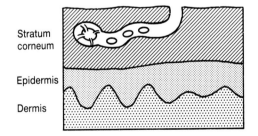

**4.61** Site of burrow in stratum corneum.

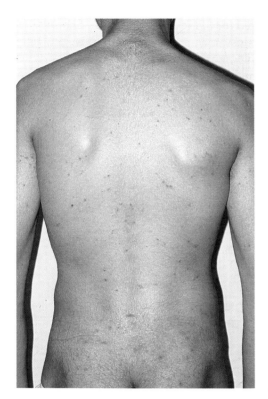

**4.62** Scabies: non-specific itchy rash affecting the whole body except the face.

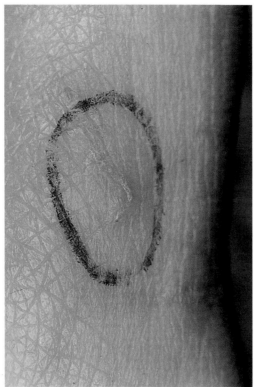

**4.63** Scabies burrow: black dot at bottom end of the burrow is where the mite is.

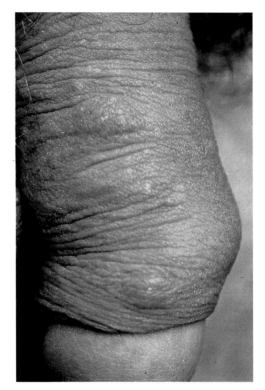

**4.64** Scabies: typical papules on penis.

The diagnosis is made by identification of the burrows which are linear S-shaped papules 3–5 mm in length usually along the sides of the fingers or on the front of the wrists. Less commonly they can be found along the sides of the feet, around the nipples, or on the buttocks or genitalia. There is almost always a rash on the hands and in males, papules on the penis and scrotum. Other members of the family or sexual partners may also be itching.

## ENDOGENOUS ECZEMA

Eczema may present as widespread itchy papules, associated with ill-defined scaly plaques. This type of rash may be indistinguishable from that found in scabies, but there will be no burrows.

## DERMATITIS HERPETIFORMIS

This is a disease of young adults and presents with severe itching particularly at night. Grouped vesicles in the distribution of psoriasis (elbows, knees, sacrum, scalp) are quickly scratched away to leave pink excoriated papules and plaques.

The diagnosis can be confirmed by biopsy of an intact blister or by finding IgA deposits in the upper dermis on immunofluorescence of normal skin. It is an important, if uncommon, disease because it is associated with a gluten enteropathy.

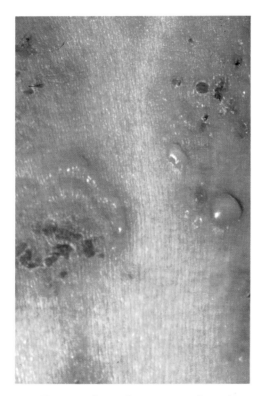

**4.65** Dermatitis herpetiformis: grouped vesicles.

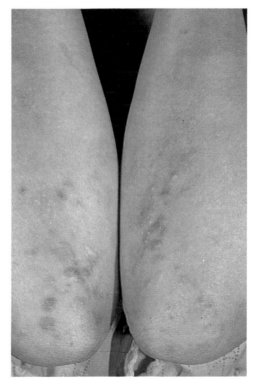

**4.66** Dermatitis herpetiformis: more usual picture with excoriated papules on elbows.

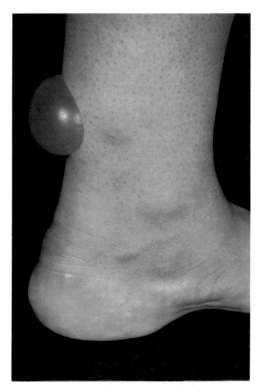

**4.67** Insect bites: occasionally large blisters can occur following insect bites. Note the ordinary bite (red papule with a central punctum) to the right of the blister.

## NODULAR PRURIGO

This is a condition in which numerous discrete intensely itchy pink, mauve or brown papules and nodules occur. They are excoriated and heal to leave white scars which sometimes have very obvious follicular openings within them.

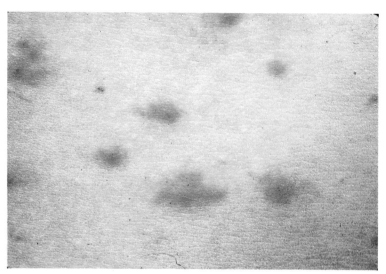

**4.69** Flea bites.

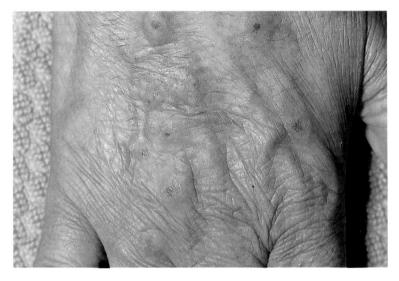

**4.68** Nodular prurigo

## INSECT BITES

Insect bites present as itchy papules with a central punctum. If there are groups or rows of 3 or 4, think of flea bites from animal fleas. Single very large lesions on the face or hands suggest bed bugs, particularly when new lesions are found each morning. Many other creatures can also bite humans.

## DERMATITIS ARTEFACTA

These lesions are self induced. The clue is that instead of being round or oval like most naturally occurring rashes they have straight sides—square, rectangular, triangular or straight lines (see Fig. 4.70). They occur anywhere the patient can reach and damage the skin with finger nails, scissors, nail files, phenol, acids, household cleaners etc. Crusting occurs from the exudate resulting from open wounds. If the lesions are occluded so that the patient cannot get at them, they normally heal very quickly. There is usually an underlying need that the patient is meeting by damaging the skin.

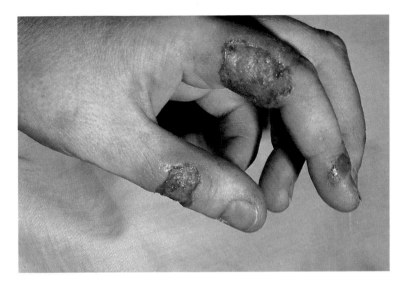

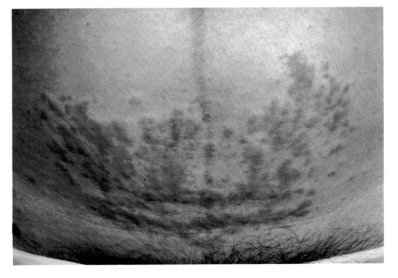

## POLYMORPHIC ERUPTION OF PREGNANCY

This condition occurs in about 1 in every 150 pregnancies and results in a rash consisting of urticated papules and vesicles. The features of this and pemphigoid gestationis are listed in Table 4.2.

**Table 4.2.** Polymorphic eruption of pregnancy and pemphigoid gestationis compared.

| Polymorphic eruption of pregnancy | Pemphigoid gestationis |
| --- | --- |
| Common (1:150) | Very rare |
| Urticated papules and vesicles | Urticated plaques → tense vesicles and bullae |
| Cause unknown | Due to autoantibody to basement membrane of skin |
| Very itchy | Very itchy |
| Usually primigravida | Once occurs, reoccurs in each subsequent pregnancy |
| Occurs 3rd trimester usually near term | Occurs 2nd and 3rd trimester |
| Clears within 2—3 weeks of delivery | Takes weeks-months to clear after delivery |
| Baby not affected | Baby may be born with same rash |

*Left above*
**4.70** Dermatitis artefacta: note square shape to lesions.

*Left below*
**4.71** Polymorphic eruption of pregnancy. This is the commonest site for the rash to start, around striae on the abdomen.

**Trunk and limbs**
**Chronic erythematous rash/lesions**
**Crusted, ulcerated or eroded surface**
**Papules, plaques or nodules**
**1  Single/few (1–5) lesions**

If crust is present, **remove** to see what is underneath

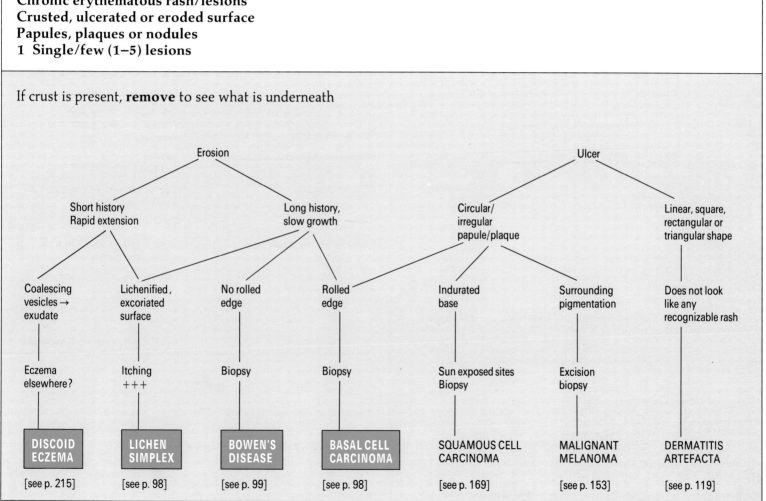

[see p. 215]   [see p. 98]   [see p. 99]   [see p. 98]   [see p. 169]   [see p. 153]   [see p. 119]

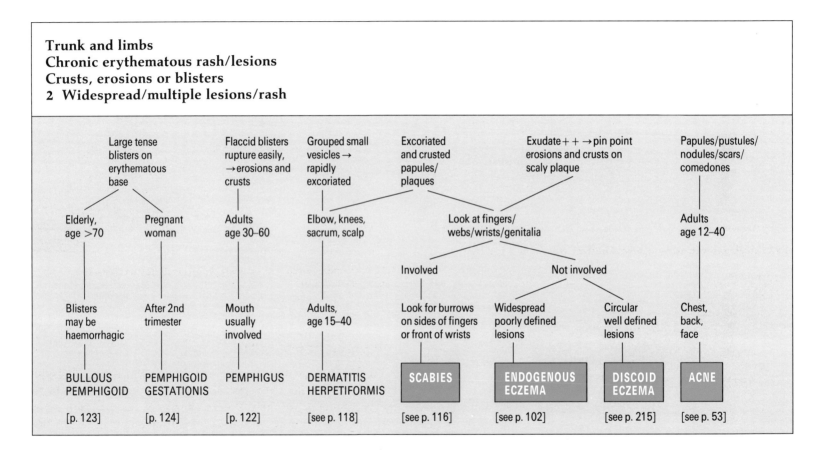

Trunk and limbs
Chronic erythematous rash/lesions
Crusts, erosions or blisters
2 Widespread/multiple lesions/rash

| Large tense blisters on erythematous base | | Flaccid blisters rupture easily, →erosions and crusts | Grouped small vesicles → rapidly excoriated | Excoriated and crusted papules/ plaques | | | Exudate++ →pin point erosions and crusts on scaly plaque | | Papules/pustules/ nodules/scars/ comedones |

| Elderly, age >70 | Pregnant woman | Adults age 30–60 | Elbow, knees, sacrum, scalp | | Look at fingers/ webs/wrists/genitalia | | | Adults age 12–40 |

| | | | | Involved | | Not involved | | |

| Blisters may be haemorrhagic | After 2nd trimester | Mouth usually involved | Adults, age 15–40 | Look for burrows on sides of fingers or front of wrists | Widespread poorly defined lesions | Circular well defined lesions | Chest, back, face |

| BULLOUS PEMPHIGOID | PEMPHIGOID GESTATIONIS | PEMPHIGUS | DERMATITIS HERPETIFORMIS | SCABIES | ENDOGENOUS ECZEMA | DISCOID ECZEMA | ACNE |

| [p. 123] | [p. 124] | [p. 122] | [see p. 118] | [see p. 116] | [see p. 102] | [see p. 215] | [see p. 53] |

## PEMPHIGUS

This is an autoimmune disease in which individual cells of the epidermis come apart from one another causing blistering (due to circulating IgG antibody localized to the intercellular substance). It is confined to the epidermis so the blisters are always very superficial, do not stay intact for very long, and form erosions and crusts. The blisters are never haemorrhagic. It often begins with erosions in the mouth and it may be weeks or months before the tell-tale blisters appear on the skin. It may spread very rapidly and be life threatening. Immediate referral to hospital is recommended.

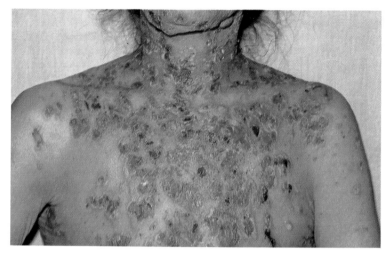

**4.72** Pemphigus: extensive superficial blisters, erosions and crusts.

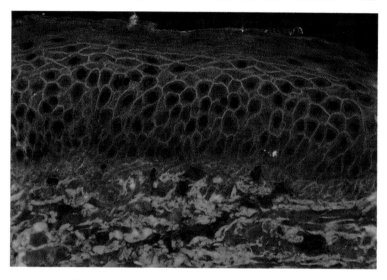

**4.74** Immunofluorescence of pemphigus: IgG antibody localized to intercellular substance.

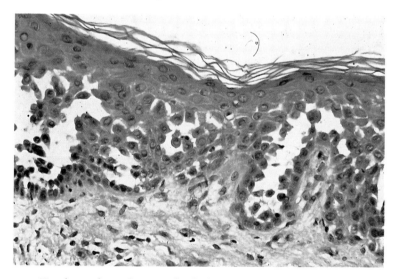

**4.73** Histology of pemphigus: individual epidermal cells have separated from each other causing a blister within the epidermis.

## BULLOUS PEMPHIGOID

Pemphigoid is another autoimmune disease which usually begins with a non-specific itchy rash that does not look quite right for either eczema or urticaria. Weeks or months later blisters occur. Here the separation of the skin is at the dermo-epidermal junction (with localization of IgG antibodies here). The roof of the blister is made up of the full thickness of the epidermis, so blisters may become large, remain intact for several days and be haemorrhagic. It is often localized to one part of the body for a while, but like pemphigus will eventually become widespread. It is the commonest cause of blisters in the elderly.

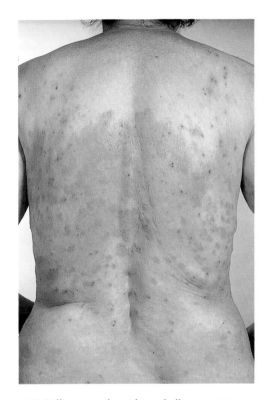

**4.75** Bullous pemphigoid: pre-bullous eruption.

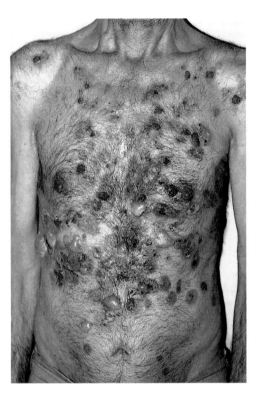

**4.76** Bullous pemphigoid: numerous large intact blisters (compare with Fig. 4.72)

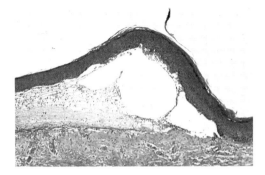

**4.77** Histology of pemphigoid: the blister occurs at the dermo-epidermal junction.

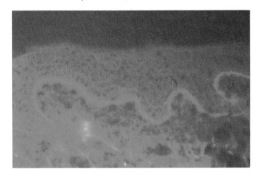

**4.78** Immunofluorescence of pemphigoid: IgG antibody localized to basement membrane of epidermis.

## PEMPHIGOID (HERPES) GESTATIONIS

This is a very rare condition occurring in pregnancy with features similar to pemphigoid; it should be differentiated from the much more common polymorphic eruption of pregnancy (see p. 120).

# Chapter 5
# Non-Erythematous Lesions on Face, Trunk and Limbs

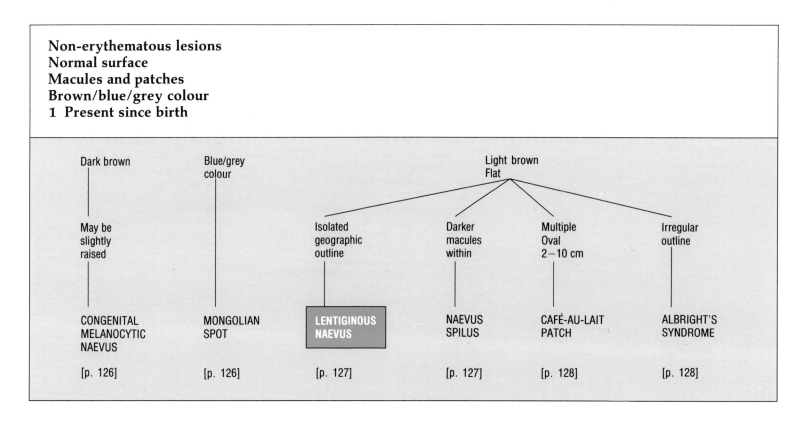

**Non-erythematous lesions**
**Normal surface**
**Macules and patches**
**Brown/blue/grey colour**
**1 Present since birth**

| Dark brown | Blue/grey colour | | Light brown Flat | | |
|---|---|---|---|---|---|
| May be slightly raised | | Isolated geographic outline | Darker macules within | Multiple Oval 2–10 cm | Irregular outline |
| CONGENITAL MELANOCYTIC NAEVUS | MONGOLIAN SPOT | LENTIGINOUS NAEVUS | NAEVUS SPILUS | CAFÉ-AU-LAIT PATCH | ALBRIGHT'S SYNDROME |
| [p. 126] | [p. 126] | [p. 127] | [p. 127] | [p. 128] | [p. 128] |

## CONGENITAL MELANOCYTIC NAEVUS

Congenital melanocytic naevi are usually larger than ordinary moles. At birth they may be red, rather than brown, but within a few months are obviously pigmented. They may be flat or raised, hairy or warty. Those bigger than 2 cm in diameter have an increased risk of malignant change: they may sometimes be very large and affect 50 percent of the body surface.

## MONGOLIAN SPOT

A large blue/grey patch on the back of an oriental baby is extremely common. It disappears spontaneously in the first year of life.

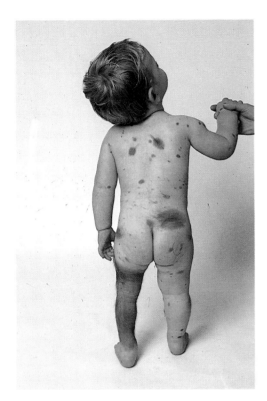

5.1 Congenital melanocytic naevus: numerous lesions in an 18 month old boy which are both pigmented and hairy.

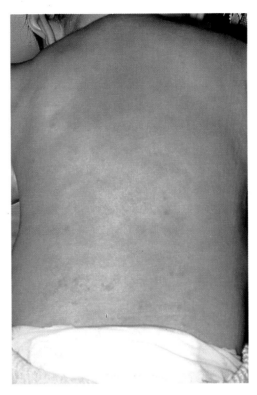

5.2 Mongolian spot.

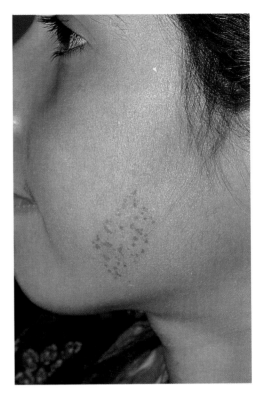

5.3 Naevus spilus.

## LENTIGINOUS NAEVUS

This is a flat pigmented birth mark, light brown in colour, oval or geographic in outline: there is no surface abnormality. It will grow with the child and remain fixed for the rest of their life.

## NAEVUS SPILUS

This is a birthmark where dark speckled macules or papules occur in a larger pigmented patch.

## CAFÉ-AU-LAIT PATCH

These are light brown patches, round or oval in shape, and often large (2−10 cm diameter). They are present at birth or appear in early childhood. If more than six are found, a diagnosis of neurofibromatosis (von Recklinghausen's disease) is likely. Look also for freckles in the axillae, multiple neurofibromas in the skin or peripheral nerves (see pp. 147, 181).

## ALBRIGHT'S SYNDROME

The full syndrome comprises irregular brown patches on the skin, fibrous dysplasia of bone presenting as pain, fractures and deformity, and precocious puberty.

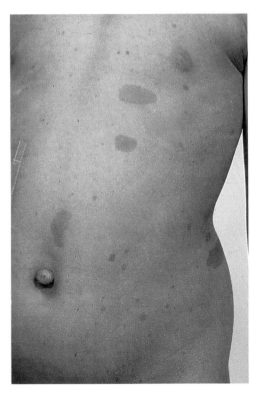

**5.4** Cafe-au-lait patches.

**Non-erythematous lesions**
**Normal/smooth surface**
**Macules and patches**
**Brown colour**
**2a  Appeared after birth—all lesions < 3 cm diameter**

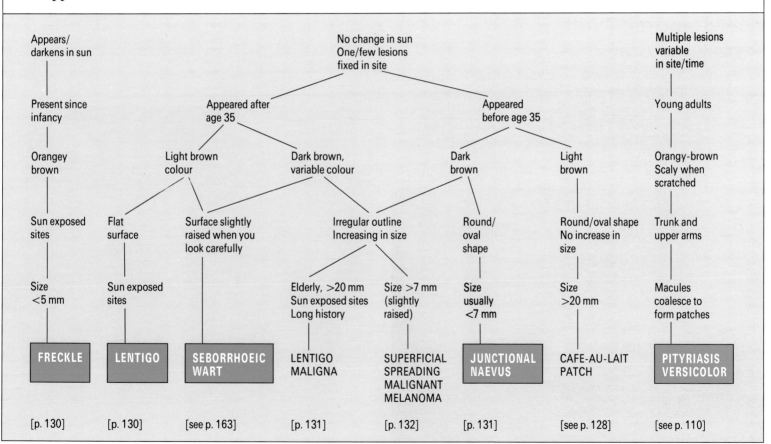

## FRECKLES (EPHELIDES)

These are small (1–5mm in diameter) orangy-brown macules which appear and increase in number and in size with sun exposure. They are commoner in red-haired, blue-eyed individuals who burn rather than tan in the sun. Histologically they contain normal numbers of melanocytes but increased melanin pigment (Fig. 5.6). They do not usually present a diagnostic problem.

## LENTIGO

Lentigoes are larger and darker than freckles and may have irregular edges. They occur mainly on sun-exposed skin but are present all the year round. Their numbers increase with increasing age: they need to be differentiated from a lentigo maligna. Histologically there are increased numbers of melanocytes in the basal layer (Fig. 5.6).

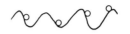

(a) Normal skin approximately 1 melanocyte/5–10 basal cells

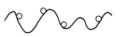

(b) Freckle same as normal skin

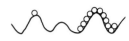

(c) Lentigo increased number of melanocytes in basal layer

5.6 Diagram to show numbers and site of melanocytes in normal skin, freckles and lentigoes.

5.7 Lentigoes on back of hand.

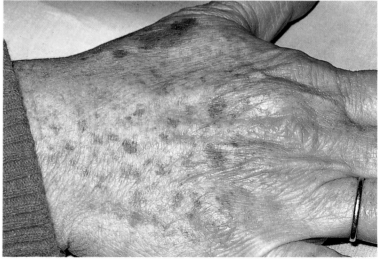

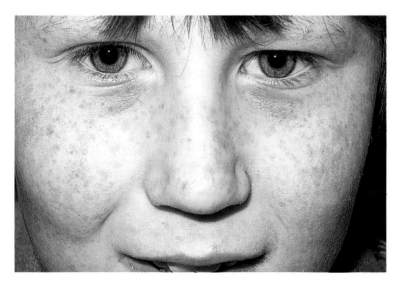

5.5 Freckles.

## LENTIGO MALIGNA (HUTCHINSON'S FRECKLE)

This looks very similar to an ordinary lentigo, but is larger (> 20 mm), has irregular edges and variation in pigment. It occurs only on sun damaged skin, most commonly on the cheeks of the elderly. It may be difficult to distinguish from a benign lentigo, but slow extension over several years is characteristic. Histologically it is a malignant melanoma confined to the epidermis (malignant melanoma-in-situ) (Fig. 5.42d, p. 153).

## JUNCTIONAL NAEVUS

A flat (sometimes slightly elevated) dark brown mole (see pp. 147, 152 for other types of moles) with regular well-defined borders. Most are smaller than 7 mm in diameter. They can occur anywhere on the skin. Histologically groups of melanocytes are found in contact with the basal layer but budding down into the dermis (Fig. 5.40, p. 152).

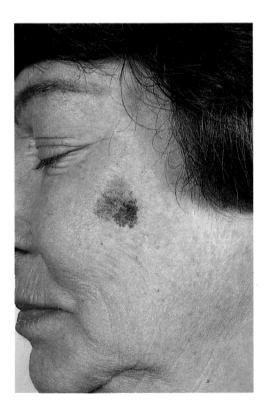

**5.8** Lentigo maligna. Compare with Fig 5.7: here the patch is larger, has a more irregular outline and greater variation in colour.

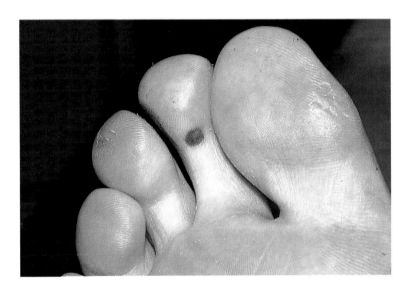

**5.9** Junctional naevus: a flat dark mole.

## SUPERFICIAL SPREADING MALIGNANT MELANOMA

The early growth phase of a malignant melanoma is horizontal with migration of the neoplastic cells outwards along the dermo-epidermal junction. This change is seen clinically as a junctional naevus enlarging in diameter, with variation in degree of pigmentation and an irregular border often with scalloped edges (see p. 153).

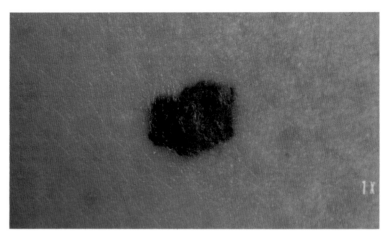

**5.11** Superficial spreading malignant melanoma. Variation in colour, irregular edge and slight scaling.

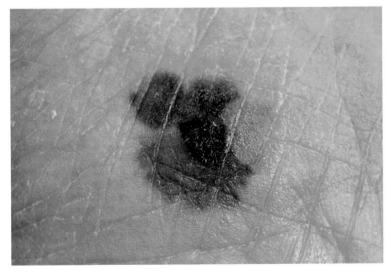

**5.10** Superficial spreading malignant melanoma. Compare with Fig 5.9: note the variation in colour and irregular edge — at this stage the skin markings are preserved.

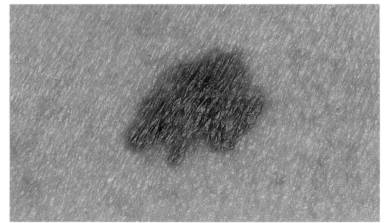

**5.12** Dysplastic naevus. Irregular edge and erythema suggestive of superficial spreading malignant melanoma clinically. This picture shows how difficult it can be to get the diagnosis right.

**Non-erythematous lesions**
**Normal surface**
**Macules and patches**
**Brown colour**
**2b  Appear after birth — some lesions > 3 cm diameter**

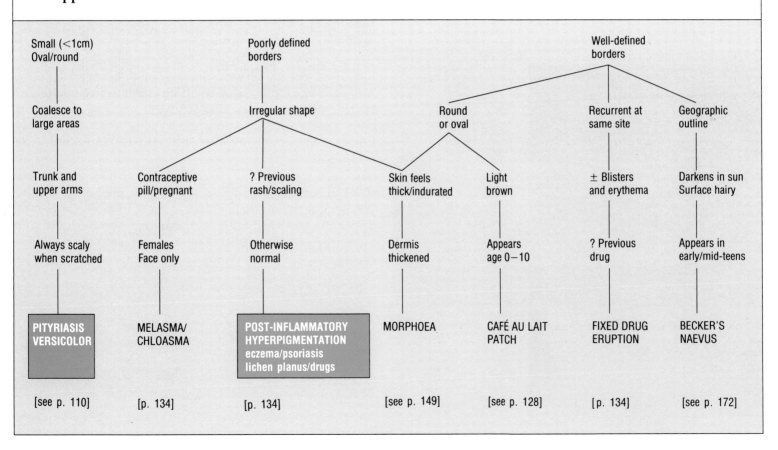

Small (<1cm) Oval/round

Coalesce to large areas

Trunk and upper arms

Always scaly when scratched

**PITYRIASIS VERSICOLOR**

[see p. 110]

Poorly defined borders

Irregular shape

Contraceptive pill/pregnant

Females Face only

MELASMA/ CHLOASMA

[p. 134]

? Previous rash/scaling

Otherwise normal

**POST-INFLAMMATORY HYPERPIGMENTATION**
eczema/psoriasis
lichen planus/drugs

[p. 134]

Round or oval

Skin feels thick/indurated

Dermis thickened

MORPHOEA

[see p. 149]

Light brown

Appears age 0–10

CAFÉ AU LAIT PATCH

[see p. 128]

Well-defined borders

Recurrent at same site

± Blisters and erythema

? Previous drug

FIXED DRUG ERUPTION

[p. 134]

Geographic outline

Darkens in sun Surface hairy

Appears in early/mid-teens

BECKER'S NAEVUS

[see p. 172]

## CHLOASMA/MELASMA

These symmetrical pigmented patches which occur in women on the forehead, cheeks and moustache area are more obvious after sun exposure. They occur most commonly during pregnancy but can be caused by the contraceptive pill, or be idiopathic. The pigmentation fades after delivery, but may be permanent. Rarely, an identical pigmentation is seen in men.

5.13 Chloasma.

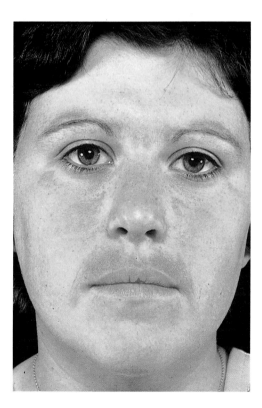

## POST-INFLAMMATORY HYPERPIGMENTATION

Macular pigmentation may follow any inflammatory process. It is commoner in darker-skinned individuals. Any involvement of the dermo-epidermal junction by disease (eczema, psoriasis, lichen planus, acne) or trauma (e.g. a burn) makes subsequent hyperpigmentation more likely. Some drugs may cause widespread pigmentation e.g. chlorpromazine, chloroquine and arsenic.

## FIXED DRUG ERUPTION

A fixed drug eruption is a round or oval inflammatory patch or plaque with or without blisters which occurs at the same site every time a particular drug is taken (usually within 2 hours following ingestion). When the redness has disappeared, a dark brown patch is left which remains for several months. Any drug can cause this but the commonest are phenolphthalein, non-steroidal anti-inflammatory drugs, sulphonamides, tetracyclines, barbiturates, various tranquillizers, and quinine (either as tablets or in tonic water and bitter lemon drinks). The diagnosis can be proved by giving the offending drug and watching the redness appear over 1–2 hours on top of the brown patch.

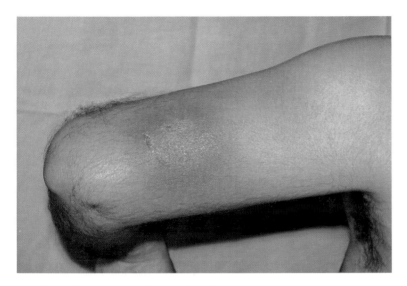

**5.14** Fixed drug eruption 3 hours after taking Septrin.

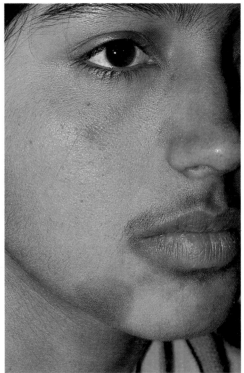

**5.16** Fixed drug eruption: brown patches left after the acute inflammation has settled. These will last for several months.

**5.15** Post inflammatory hyperpigmentation.

## Non-erythematous lesions
## Surface normal/smooth
## Macules and/or patches
## White colour

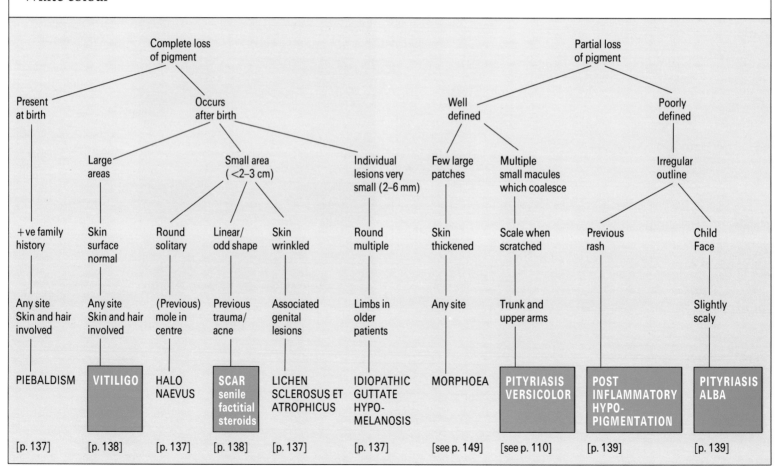

## PIEBALDISM

This is an inherited condition (autosomal dominant) where patches of complete depigmentation are present at birth, and remain unchanged throughout life. It may be associated with a white forelock of hair if the skin in that area is affected. Clinically it is identical to vitiligo which develops later in life.

## LICHEN SCLEROSUS ET ATROPHICUS

This condition usually presents with genital itching and is seen as white atrophic plaques in the perineum. Rarely the trunk and limbs may also be involved: small flat white atrophic macules and papules with a shiny wrinkled surface occur, most commonly on the upper trunk (see p. 279).

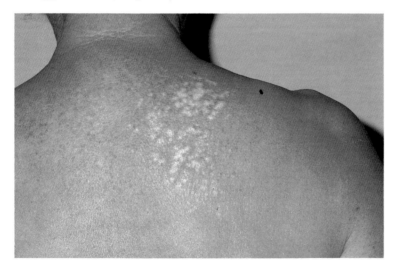

5.17 Lichen sclerosus et atrophicus on the back. Patient also has involvement of vulva.

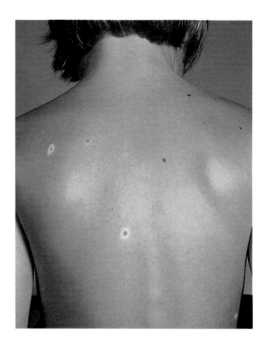

5.18 Two halo naevi on back.

## HALO NAEVUS

An immunological reaction against melanocytes in a mole produces a halo of depigmentation around the mole. Eventually the mole disappears. This reaction is quite benign and does not indicate that the mole has undergone malignant change.

## IDIOPATHIC GUTTATE HYPOMELANOSIS

Small (2–6 mm) white macules appear on sun-exposed parts of the limbs in the middle-aged and elderly. They have well-defined borders and normal skin markings, and are due to localized sun damage to melanocytes.

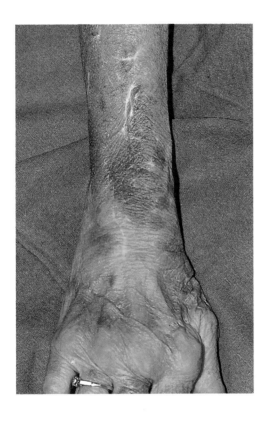

**5.19** Odd shaped scars on forearm due to tearing of skin after minor trauma. Patient had been using potent topical steroids on the skin. Note also the purpura from the same cause.

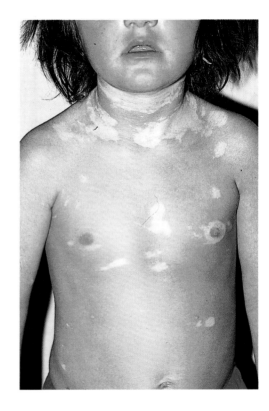

**5.20** Vitiligo in an Iranian child

## SCARRING

Scars may be flat or raised: usually the patient will remember the cause. Scars due to an injury or operation are linear; those with odd shapes may be due to self-inflicted damage; those that are crescent shaped or star shaped may be due to tearing of the skin after minor trauma in patients taking oral corticosteroids or using potent topical steroids. Normal degrees of itching and scratching do not lead to scarring.

## VITILIGO

Vitiligo is caused by idiopathic loss of melanocytes from the skin. It consists of well-defined white patches in normal skin. Usually there are few, large, irregular-shaped patches rather than multiple small macules. The hair in the depigmented areas may also be depigmented. The condition is slowly progressive, although it may remain static or even show areas of repigmentation. It is obviously more noticeable in patients with dark skins for whom it may be a gross cosmetic disability. There may be areas of hyper-pigmentation around the edge of a white patch, and very fair-skinned individuals may complain of the hyperpigmentation rather than the hypopigmentation. The affected areas burn easily when exposed to sunlight. Histologically there is an absence of melanocytes. Vitiligo may be associated with organ-specific auto-immune diseases such as hypo- and hyperthyroidism, pernicious anaemia, Addison's disease and diabetes mellitis.

On the trunk it is often confused with pityriasis versicolor (see p. 110).

## POST-INFLAMMATORY HYPOPIGMENTATION

Partial loss of pigment may follow any inflammatory skin condition, just as some individuals will produce hyperpigmentation in response to the same stimulus. It is distinguished from pityriasis

versicolor in being more ill-defined and irregular in outline, and producing little or no scale on scratching the surface.

## PITYRIASIS ALBA

Multiple, poorly-defined, hypopigmented, slightly scaly patches can occur on the face of children. In Caucasians they may only be visible in the summer when the normal skin tans. In dark skinned individuals it is relatively common. It is considered to be a mild form of eczema.

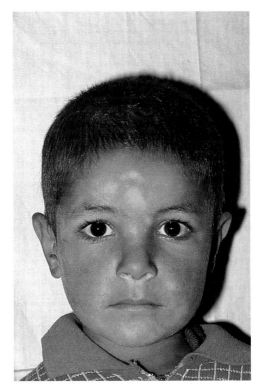

*Left*
**5.21** Post-inflammatory hypo- and hyperpigmentation following discoid lupus erythematosus.

*Right*
**5.22** Pityriasis alba.

**Non-erythematous lesions**
**Normal/smooth surface**
**Small papules (< 5 mm in size)**
**1 Skin coloured/light pink/yellow**

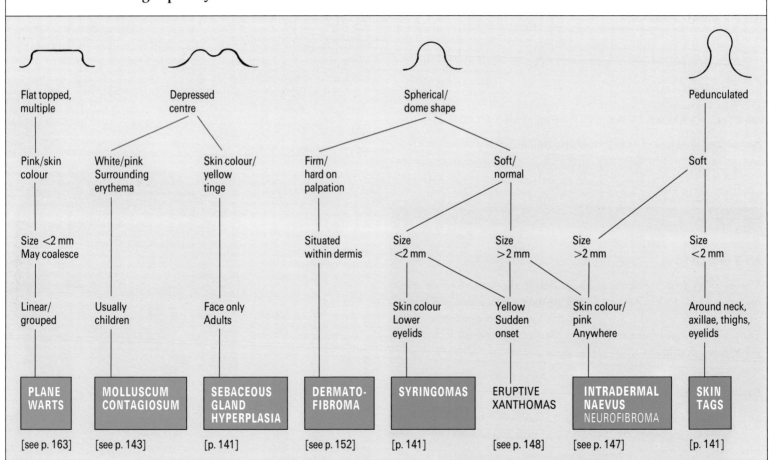

| Flat topped, multiple | Depressed centre | | Spherical/ dome shape | | | Pedunculated |
|---|---|---|---|---|---|---|
| Pink/skin colour | White/pink Surrounding erythema | Skin colour/ yellow tinge | Firm/ hard on palpation | Soft/ normal | | Soft |
| Size <2 mm May coalesce | | | Situated within dermis | Size <2 mm | Size >2 mm | Size >2 mm | Size <2 mm |
| Linear/ grouped | Usually children | Face only Adults | | Skin colour Lower eyelids | Yellow Sudden onset | Skin colour/ pink Anywhere | Around neck, axillae, thighs, eyelids |
| **PLANE WARTS** | **MOLLUSCUM CONTAGIOSUM** | **SEBACEOUS GLAND HYPERPLASIA** | **DERMATO-FIBROMA** | **SYRINGOMAS** | ERUPTIVE XANTHOMAS | **INTRADERMAL NAEVUS** NEUROFIBROMA | **SKIN TAGS** |
| [see p. 163] | [see p. 143] | [p. 141] | [see p. 152] | [p. 141] | [see p. 148] | [see p. 147] | [p. 141] |

## SEBACEOUS GLAND HYPERPLASIA

This is a benign lesion which may sometimes cause diagnostic confusion with an early basal cell carcinoma. It is usually yellowish rather than translucent in colour and consists of a small papule, 2–5 mm in diameter, with a central punctum which gives the edge a rolled appearance.

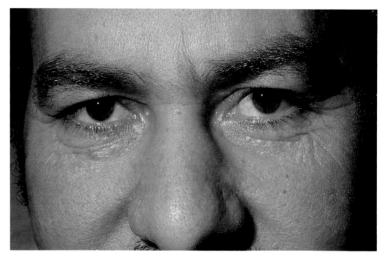

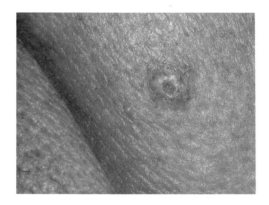

**5.23** Sebaceous gland hyperplasia (compare with Fig. 5.30).

## SYRINGOMA

These differ from xanthelasmas in being skin coloured or translucent, round in shape and small in size (1–5 mm). They most commonly occur symmetrically on the lower eyelids after puberty. They are benign tumours of sweat glands and are inherited as an autosomal dominant trait.

**5.24** Multiple syringomas below the eyes.

## SKIN TAGS

Skin tags are small, pedunculated, skin-coloured or brown papules around the neck, in the axillae, and sometimes on the upper thighs.

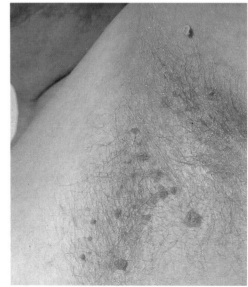

**5.25** Skin tags.

**Non-erythematous lesions**
**Normal/smooth surface**
**Small papules (< 5 mm size)**
**2  White/cream coloured**

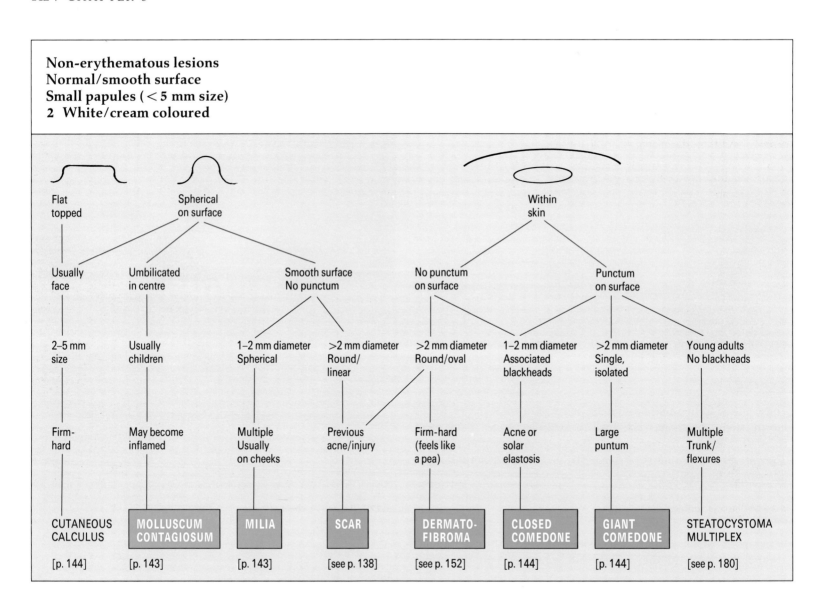

| Flat topped | Spherical on surface | | | Within skin | | | |
|---|---|---|---|---|---|---|---|
| Usually face | Umbilicated in centre | Smooth surface No punctum | | No punctum on surface | | Punctum on surface | |
| 2–5 mm size | Usually children | 1–2 mm diameter Spherical | >2 mm diameter Round/ linear | >2 mm diameter Round/oval | 1–2 mm diameter Associated blackheads | >2 mm diameter Single, isolated | Young adults No blackheads |
| Firm-hard | May become inflamed | Multiple Usually on cheeks | Previous acne/injury | Firm-hard (feels like a pea) | Acne or solar elastosis | Large puntum | Multiple Trunk/ flexures |
| CUTANEOUS CALCULUS | MOLLUSCUM CONTAGIOSUM | MILIA | SCAR | DERMATO-FIBROMA | CLOSED COMEDONE | GIANT COMEDONE | STEATOCYSTOMA MULTIPLEX |
| [p. 144] | [p. 143] | [p. 143] | [see p. 138] | [see p. 152] | [p. 144] | [p. 144] | [see p. 180] |

## MOLLUSCUM CONTAGIOSUM

This is a viral infection (poxvirus) of the skin usually affecting children. Small 1–5 mm white or pink umbilicated papules are found anywhere on the skin and there may be few or many. They can become inflamed and red in colour. They last about 6–9 months and then disappear spontaneously.

They are sometimes confused with viral warts because both occur in children, but they look quite different (compare Figs. 5.26, 5.56 and 8.18, pp. 143, 162 and 222).

## MILIA

These are very small superficial epidermoid cysts. They are 1–2 mm in diameter, white, spherical papules protruding above the surface of the skin on the cheeks and eyelids. They can occur spontaneously or follow any acute subepidermal blister, e.g. after burns, or other blistering diseases.

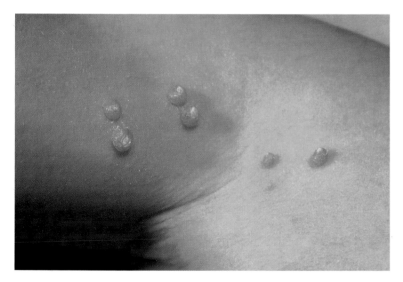

**5.26** Molluscum contagiosum.

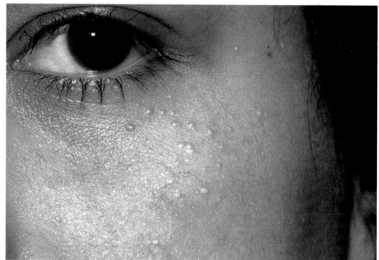

**5.27** Milia on the cheek.

## CUTANEOUS CALCULUS

These are single, white, round, flat-topped papules on the face of a child, and they feel firm to hard on palpation. They are harmless and made up of calcium deposited in the upper dermis.

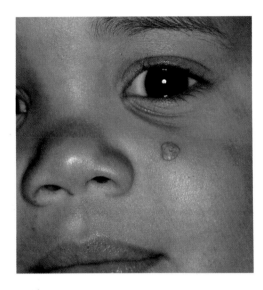

**5.28** Cutaneous calculus.

## GIANT COMEDONE

Single large comedones can occur on the trunk and face in the elderly. They are much larger than the blackheads associated with acne in teenagers, but the aetiology is basically the same; a single follicle with a keratin plug at its mouth, filling up with keratin and sebum behind it. Clinically it is a white/cream papule with a central black punctum.

## CLOSED COMEDONE

A comedone is a single blocked pilosebaceous follicle. The opening in a closed comedone (whitehead) is not obvious; keratin, sebum, and hair fragments accumulate within the follicle to produce a spherical white papule. It is usually within the skin with only the most superficial part protruding above the surface. Closed comedones are associated with open comedones (blackheads) in teenagers and young adults with acne vulgaris (see Fig. 3.29, p. 53). In the elderly, similar lesions occur in areas of solar elastosis around the eyes or on the cheeks.

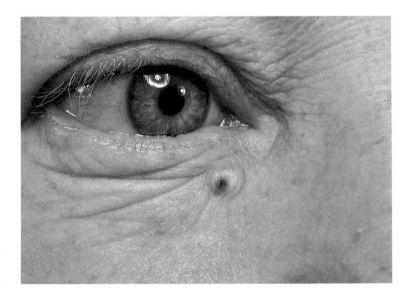

**5.29** Giant comedone.

**Non-erythematous lesions**
**Normal/smooth surface**
**Large papules (> 5 mm), plaques and nodules**
**Skin coloured/white/cream/yellow/pink**
**1 Situated on surface of skin**          ⎰⎱ or ⌒ shape

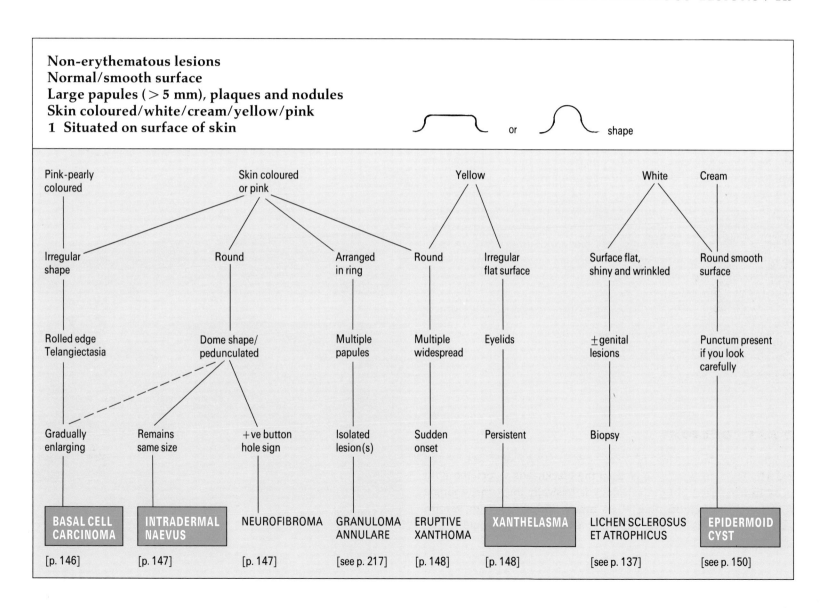

| Pink-pearly coloured | Skin coloured or pink | | | Yellow | | White | Cream |
|---|---|---|---|---|---|---|---|
| Irregular shape | Round | Arranged in ring | Round | Irregular flat surface | Surface flat, shiny and wrinkled | Round smooth surface |
| Rolled edge Telangiectasia | Dome shape/ pedunculated | Multiple papules | Multiple widespread | Eyelids | ±genital lesions | Punctum present if you look carefully |
| Gradually enlarging | Remains same size | +ve button hole sign | Isolated lesion(s) | Sudden onset | Persistent | Biopsy |
| **BASAL CELL CARCINOMA** | **INTRADERMAL NAEVUS** | NEUROFIBROMA | GRANULOMA ANNULARE | ERUPTIVE XANTHOMA | **XANTHELASMA** | LICHEN SCLEROSUS ET ATROPHICUS | **EPIDERMOID CYST** |
| [p. 146] | [p. 147] | [p. 147] | [see p. 217] | [p. 148] | [p. 148] | [see p. 137] | [see p. 150] |

## BASAL CELL CARCINOMA (RODENT ULCER)

This is the commonest malignant tumour of the skin. It usually occurs on exposed areas in people who have had a lot of sun exposure in the past, and is most common in those with red hair, blue eyes and freckles. Although due to ultraviolet light, it does not occur at sites of maximum sun exposure, i.e. it rarely occurs on the bald scalp, ears, lower lips or backs of hands (sites where squamous cell carcinomas are more common).

A basal cell carcinoma starts as a small papule, pink or pearly in colour usually with obvious telangiectasia over the surface. This gradually enlarges to a nodule or by circumferential growth to produce a flatter lesion (it may only reach a diameter of 1 cm over about 5 years). It is most important to look carefully at the border which tends to be rolled and raised above the centre, like a piece of string around the edge. It may be necessary to stretch the skin to see this in a very flat lesion. The centre often breaks down forming an ulcer, which may be covered with a serous or blood stained crust.

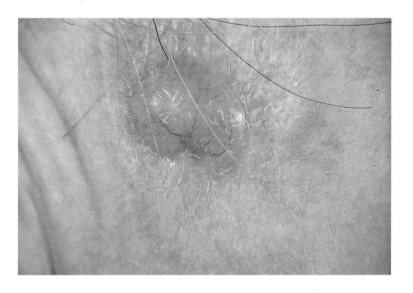

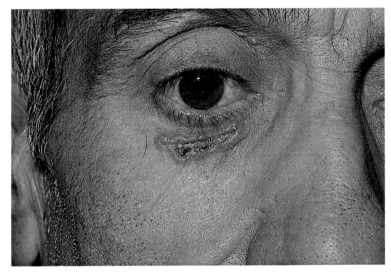

*Right above*
**5.30** Basal cell carcinoma. Early lesion not yet ulcerated: note translucent appearance and telangiectasia.

*Right below*
**5.31** Basal cell carcinoma: typical rolled edge with ulceration and crusting in the centre.

## INTRADERMAL NAEVUS

This is a skin coloured mole; the naevus cells have all dropped into the dermis so the pigment is no longer seen on the surface (see Fig. 5.40, p. 152). The individual lesions are small, round, dome-shaped or papillomatous papules. Occasionally telangiectasia can be seen on the surface, but the lack of growth, long history and symmetrical shape of the lesion distinguish it from a basal cell carcinoma.

They are sometimes pedunculated, and can be difficult to distinguish from neurofibromas or skin tags; if in doubt excision and histological examination will give the answer.

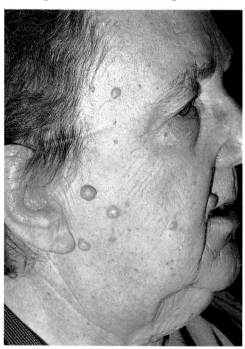

**5.32** Multiple intradermal naevi: raised skin coloured moles.

## NEUROFIBROMA

These are skin-coloured, pink or red tumours derived from peripheral nerves. If you press the surface, the papules are usually soft and often a hole can be felt in the bottom (like the hole in a button). They can be solitary, or multiple when they are associated with café-au-lait patches (von Recklinghausen's disease). Isolated lesions may be indistinguishable clinically from intradermal naevi.

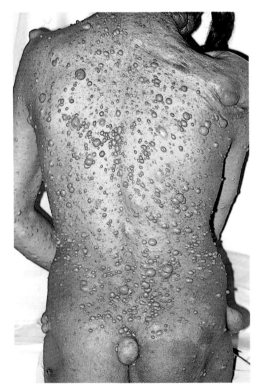

**5.33** Neurofibromatosis (von Recklinghausen's disease). Multiple neurofibromas of all shapes and sizes with two cafe-au-lait patches on the right buttock.

## ERUPTIVE XANTHOMA

Eruptive xanthomas are yellow papules containing lipid deposits secondary to hyperlipidaemia. The lesions clear once the triglyceride levels return to normal.

## XANTHELASMA

These are yellow flat plaques usually found on the eyelids. They are not necessarily associated with hyperlipidaemia, but xanthelasmas are more common in patients with atherosclerosis.

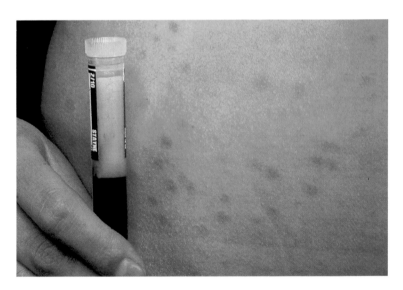

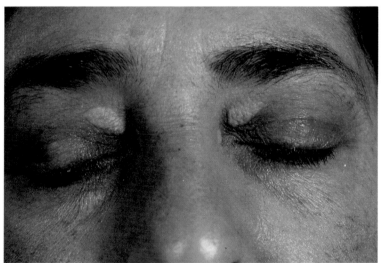

**5.34** Eruptive xanthomas on the buttock and the patient's blood showing the hyperlipidaemia.

**5.35** Xanthelasmas on both upper eyelids.

**Non-erythematous lesions
Normal surface
Skin coloured/white/cream/yellow/light pink
Papules (> 5mm), plaques and nodules
2b Situated deep**

```
              Irregular                              Spherical
              shape                                  shape


    Skin thickened  Mobile           Fixed to              Present
    and indurated   under skin       overlying skin        from birth


    Purple          No               Central   No punctum  Central punctum
    border          punctum          punctum   < 1 cm      ± hairs protruding


                    Soft/            ± Previous  Firm–      ± Previous
                    firm             inflammation hard      inflammation


    MORPHOEA      LIPOMA    EPIDERMOID  DERMATO-   DERMOID CYST
                            CYST        FIBROMA

    [p. 149]      [p. 150]  [p. 150]  [see p. 152]  [p. 150]
```

## MORPHOEA

This is a localized thickening of the dermis with excessive collagen and loss of appendages (sweat glands and hair follicles). It occurs at any age (peak incidence from 20–40), and is more common in females. The lesion is a firm oval plaque with a shiny smooth surface. The edge is often purple or brown while the centre is white or yellow. It feels thickened compared to the surrounding skin. Rarely it may be linear going down an arm or leg, or on the forehead ('en coup de sabre'). Localized lesions tend to resolve spontaneously. In rare instances, morphoea can be extensive, and when involving large areas of the chest wall breathing may be impeded. It is not related to systemic sclerosis, which is a widespread multi-system disease.

**5.36** Morphoea.

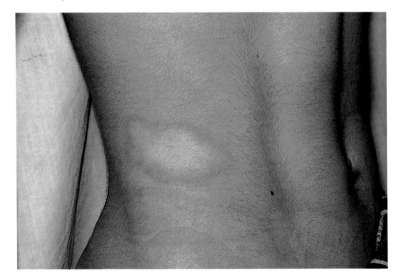

## LIPOMA

This is a benign tumour of fat cells presenting as a soft or firm subcutaneous nodule, round or irregular in shape. Nodules may be single or multiple and vary in size from ½–10cm in diameter. The overlying skin is normal. Usually they are of no significance. They need to be distinguished from epidermoid cysts.

## EPIDERMOID CYST

This is a well-circumscribed papule or nodule situated within the dermis. It is commonly misnamed a 'sebaceous cyst', but the lining of the cyst looks like normal epidermis and it is derived from the upper part of the external root sheath of a hair follicle or from a sweat duct. The cheesy material within the cyst is altered keratin produced by the epidermal lining. Usually a central punctum marking the opening of the hair follicle is visible, and through this the cyst contents may become secondarily infected. Once this has occurred they become difficult to enucleate.

They are inherited as an autosomal dominant trait but appear after puberty (usually 15–30 years). If epidermoid cysts occur before puberty they may be associated with polyposis coli. Similar cysts may occur in patients with acne after damage to hair follicles, or after penetrating injuries where bits of epidermis are implanted into the dermis.

*Gardner's Syndrome*

## DERMOID CYST

These look like epidermoid cysts but have been present from birth or early childhood. They are due to inclusion of epidermis and its appendages in the dermis at the time of embryonic skin closure. Most occur on the head and neck, either in the midline or at the lateral end of the eyebrow.

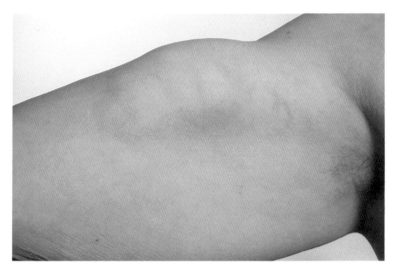

**5.37** Lipoma.

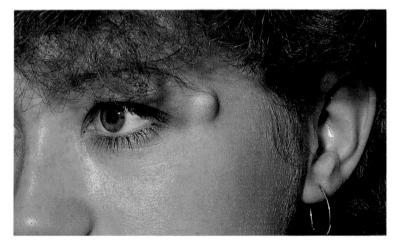

**5.38** Epidermoid cyst, appeared at age 20.

# Non-erythematous lesions
## Surface normal
## Papules, plaques and nodules
## Brown colour

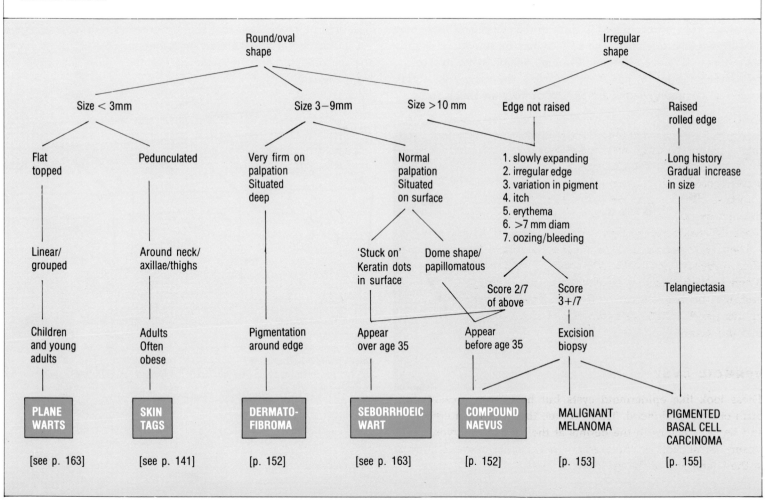

Round/oval shape
Irregular shape

Size < 3mm | Size 3–9mm | Size >10 mm | Edge not raised | Raised rolled edge

Flat topped
Pedunculated
Very firm on palpation Situated deep
Normal palpation Situated on surface
1. slowly expanding
2. irregular edge
3. variation in pigment
4. itch
5. erythema
6. >7 mm diam
7. oozing/bleeding
Long history Gradual increase in size

Linear/ grouped
Around neck/ axillae/thighs
'Stuck on' Keratin dots in surface
Dome shape/ papillomatous
Telangiectasia

Score 2/7 of above
Score 3+/7

Children and young adults
Adults Often obese
Pigmentation around edge
Appear over age 35
Appear before age 35
Excision biopsy

**PLANE WARTS**
**SKIN TAGS**
**DERMATO-FIBROMA**
**SEBORRHOEIC WART**
**COMPOUND NAEVUS**
MALIGNANT MELANOMA
PIGMENTED BASAL CELL CARCINOMA

[see p. 163] | [see p. 141] | [p. 152] | [see p. 163] | [p. 152] | [p. 153] | [p. 155]

## DERMATOFIBROMA (HISTIOCYTOMA)

This is a firm—hard papule situated in the dermis and occurs anywhere on the body. It is often due to trauma or an insect bite, so is commonly found on ladies' legs. It is often small (< 1cm), attached to the skin and mobile over deeper structures. The colour can range from skin coloured to pink in the centre and there may be a brown circumference. The surface may be smooth or slightly scaly. Once developed dermatofibromas remain static in size.

Provided the lesion has been palpated, the diagnosis is easy since few common lesions are as hard; moles are much softer.

**5.39** Dermatofibroma. Note the pigment in a ring at the edge of the papule.

## COMPOUND NAEVUS

These are raised brown moles with a rounded or papillamatous surface. The natural history of moles is a maturation from junctional naevi (flat and dark brown) to compound naevi (brown papules) to intradermal naevi (skin coloured papules), see Fig. 5.40. It should be recognized that this progression in a mole is *normal benign* change and not a sign of malignant change. In fact once the melanocytes drop into the dermis they loose any potential for malignant change.

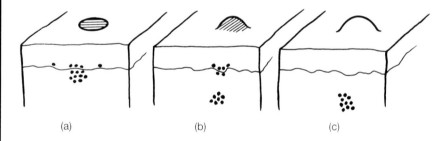

(a)  (b)  (c)

**5.40** Histological features of melanocytic naevi.
(a) Junctional naevus: flat, brown round/oval lesion. Melanocytes at dermo-epidermal junction.
(b) Compound naevus: raised, brown papule. Melanocytes at dermo-epidermal junction *and* intradermally.
(c) Intradermal naevus: raised, skin coloured papule. All melanocytes intradermal.

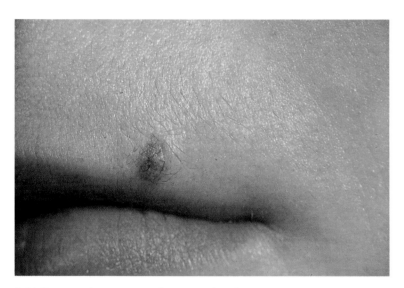

5.41 Compound naevus: raised pigmented mole.

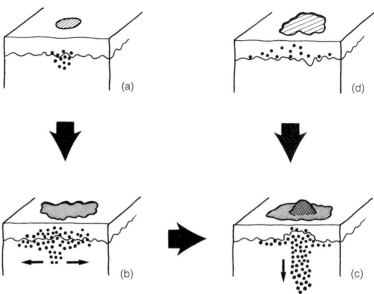

## MALIGNANT MELANOMA

A malignant melanoma is a malignant tumour of melanocytes. 50 per cent arise from a pre-existing mole which has junctional activity (i.e. a junctional or compound naevus); the other half arise out of normal skin. The initial phase of growth of the melanoma is horizontal along the junction of epidermis and dermis, and is manifest clinically as a superficial spreading melanoma (Fig. 5.42). This type of lesion is flat or only slightly raised (see p. 132) Later (months – years) vertical growth occurs with the melanoma cells invading deeper into the dermis, coming into contact with blood vessels and lymphatics so that metastatic spread is more likely. Clinically the lesion becomes more raised, and the surface may break down with exudation, crusting or bleeding.

There is a direct correlation between the thickness of a melanoma

5.42 Development of malignant melanoma from a mole.
(a) Junctional naevus: melanocytes at dermo-epidermal junction
(b) Superficial spreading melanoma: malignant cells migrate horizontally. Prognosis good.
(c) Nodular malignant melanoma: malignant cell migrate vertically and can invade lymphatics. Prognosis poor.
(d) Lentigo maligna: abnormal melanocytes restricted to epidermis. Prognosis good.

(Breslow thickness—from top of granular layer to deepest point of invasion) and prognosis as measured by survival rates (Fig. 5.45). It is therefore important that malignant melanomas should be diagnosed and removed as early as possible when they are in the horizontal growth phase.

To help in the diagnosis of malignant versus benign moles, a 7

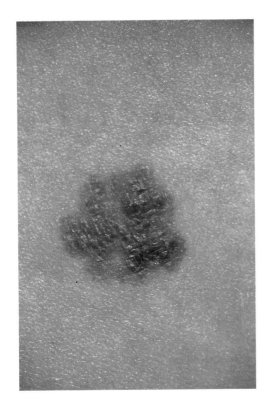

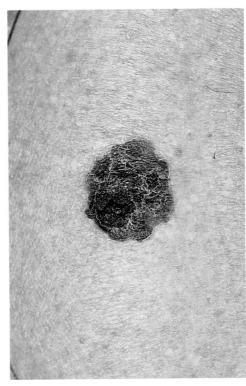

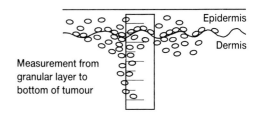

Measurement from
granular layer to
bottom of tumour

Epidermis

Dermis

% survival at 5 years

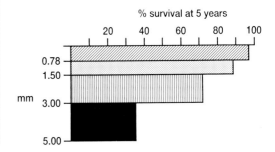

**5.43** Superficial spreading malignant melanoma: note the erythema and irregular edge.

**5.44** Superficial spreading malignant melanoma: note the colour variation, irregular edge and surface scaling.

**5.45** Prognosis of malignant melanoma related to Breslow thickness.

point check list has been devised (Table 5.1). If 2 or less of the features described are present then one can be confident that a mole is benign. If 3 or more features are present then an urgent referral to a dermatologist, or excision of the whole lesion with histological examination is necessary.

Malignant melanomas need to be differentiated from compound naevi (p. 152), blue naevi (p. 157), irritated seborrhoeic warts (p. 159) and pyogenic granulomas (p. 160).

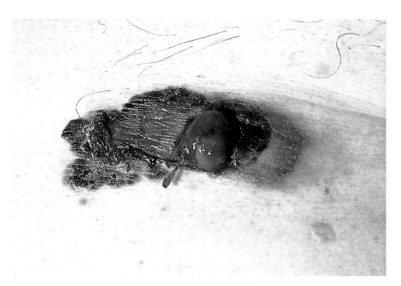

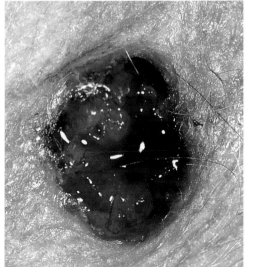

**Table 5.1.** Check list of clinical features found in melanomas.
2 or less, the mole is benign; 3 or more refer for biopsy (courtesy Prof R. M. MacKie, Glasgow University)

1   **Itch**. Benign moles do not itch, malignant ones may.

2   **Size > 1 cm**. Most malignant lesions have reached 1 cm in diameter before they are recognized, while benign lesions are usually smaller.

3   **Increasing size**. Malignant lesions increase in diameter, while benign lesions may become more elevated but should never increase in diameter.

4   **Irregular outline**. Benign lesions have a round or oval shape, while malignant lesions have a scalloped or notched border.

5   **Colour variation**. Malignant lesions usually show variation in colour from black to light brown, and may even have a reddish tint due to inflammation.

6   **Inflammation**. Benign lesions should never have any evidence of erythema within or around the margin of the lesion.

7   **Crusting/oozing/bleeding**. Can occur in a malignant lesion and may be the reason why the patient has consulted the doctor.

5.46 Nodular malignant melanoma.

5.47 Pigmented basal cell carcinoma: compare rolled edge with that in Fig. 5.31.

## PIGMENTED BASAL CELL CARCINOMA

Occasionally a basal cell carcinoma is heavily pigmented and can be confused with a nodular malignant melanoma, but the typical rolled edge should suggest the diagnosis (see p. 146).

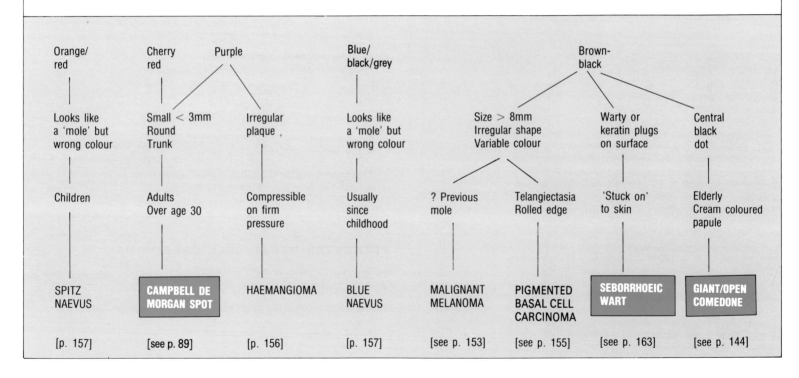

Non-erythematous/erythematous lesions
Normal surface
Papules, plaques and nodules
Blue/black/purple/red/orange colour
1 No recent increase in size

| Orange/red | Cherry red | Purple | Blue/black/grey | | Brown-black | | |
|---|---|---|---|---|---|---|---|
| Looks like a 'mole' but wrong colour | Small < 3mm Round Trunk | Irregular plaque | Looks like a 'mole' but wrong colour | Size > 8mm Irregular shape Variable colour | | Warty or keratin plugs on surface | Central black dot |
| Children | Adults Over age 30 | Compressible on firm pressure | Usually since childhood | ? Previous mole | Telangiectasia Rolled edge | 'Stuck on' to skin | Elderly Cream coloured papule |
| SPITZ NAEVUS | CAMPBELL DE MORGAN SPOT | HAEMANGIOMA | BLUE NAEVUS | MALIGNANT MELANOMA | PIGMENTED BASAL CELL CARCINOMA | SEBORRHOEIC WART | GIANT/OPEN COMEDONE |
| [p. 157] | [see p. 89] | [p. 156] | [p. 157] | [see p. 153] | [see p. 155] | [see p. 163] | [see p. 144] |

## HAEMANGIOMA

Purple papules and plaques which have been present since childhood are due to a localized overgrowth of blood vessels. The stagnant blood within the lesion may be compressed partially, but the colour will never fade completely. Haemangiomas vary in size, and may occur at any time during childhood.

## SPITZ NAEVUS

These look like moles but they are red or orange in colour. In children they cannot be mistaken for anything else. They are not common in adults and if they are removed the histology is found to be very similar to a malignant melanoma, sometimes causing some anxiety: they are however benign.

## BLUE NAEVUS

These look like moles but are dark blue or black in colour. They are slightly raised and usually less than 10 mm in diameter. They appear during childhood and then remain fixed, a feature which will distinguish them from a malignant melanoma.

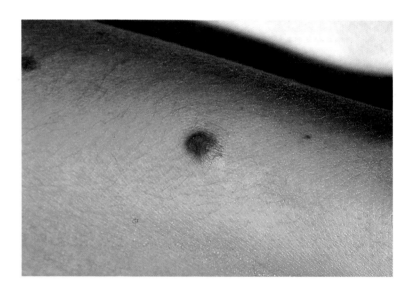

**5.49** Blue naevus.

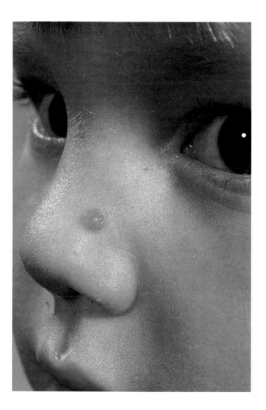

**5.48** Spitz naevus.

**Non-erythematous/erythematous lesions**
**Normal/smooth surface**
**Papules and nodules**
**Blue/black/red/purple colour**
**2 Recent increase in size**

Onset age
1 week to 1 month

Onset after
age 1 month

Usually
single

Single
lesion

Single/multiple
lesion(s)

Irregular
shape

Round
shape

Purple/pink/
red/brown

Rapid growth
up to age
12–15 months

Surrounding
pigmentation

Not bled

Bled after trauma/
spontaneously

Initially macule
→papule/nodule

Diascopy: pigment
irregular/darker
at the edge

Diascopy:
dilated blood
vessels seen

Trauma to
previous
lesion

No previous
lesion

HIV +ve

STRAWBERRY
NAEVUS

MALIGNANT
MELANOMA

THROMBOSED
HAEMANGIOMA

**IRRITATED
SEBORRHOEIC
WART**

**PYOGENIC
GRANULOMA**

KAPOSI'S
SARCOMA

[p. 159]

[see p. 153]

[see p. 156]

[p. 159]

[p. 160]

[p. 160]

## STRAWBERRY NAEVUS

These red nodules are quite unmistakable. They are not present at birth but appear usually between the 1st and 4th week of life. They grow quite quickly up to the age of 12–15 months, and then gradually and spontaneously involute. During this phase the colour becomes more purple, and as the nodule shrinks the overlying skin becomes slightly flaccid. Most lesions resolve completely by the age of 7 but may leave some residual flaccidity of the skin. The main problem is a cosmetic one, but if traumatized, haemorrhage and ulceration can occur. Rarely platelet consumption (Kasbach-Merritt syndrome) can occur causing thrombocytopenia.

## IRRITATED SEBORRHOEIC WART

A seborrhoeic wart may be caught in clothing, half torn off and become red and inflamed. It may then be easily mistaken for a mole that has undergone malignant change and result in the patient consulting the doctor. The lesion usually has the 'stuck on' appearance of the original lesion, but will have surrounding erythema rather than pigmentation. If the diagnosis is in doubt, it should be removed for histological examination.

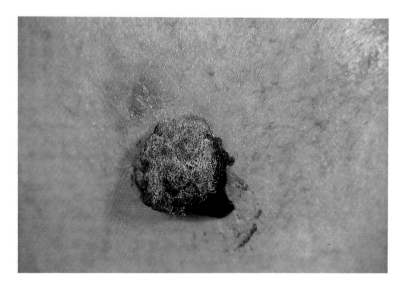

**5.51** Irritated seborrhoeic wart: it has been caught in the patient's clothes and partly torn off, hence the bleeding.

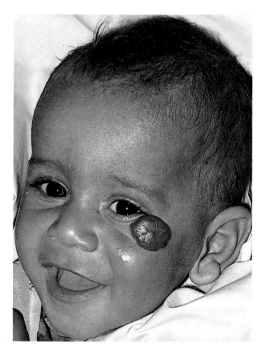

**5.50** Strawberry naevus.

## PYOGENIC GRANULOMA

This is due to localized overgrowth of blood vessels in response to trauma, often a graze or prick. There is very rapid growth over a few weeks, and usually a history of the lesion having bled spontaneously at some stage. The lesion will be round in shape, bright red or purple in colour, and the surrounding skin will be quite normal. In contrast, an amelanotic malignant melanoma usually is irregular in shape, has some surrounding pigmentation and grows over a period of months rather than days or weeks.

## KAPOSI'S SARCOMA

This is malignant growth of blood vessels which was previously rare, but is now seen in patients with AIDS. The lesions begin as small purple-red, reddish-brown or purple macules or papules. They may grow quite quickly and become nodular or form plaques. Screening for HIV titres and biopsy are necessary for diagnosis.

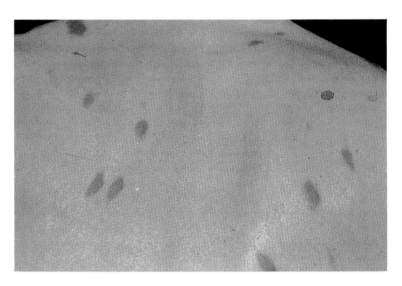

**5.53** Kaposi's sarcoma in a patient with AIDS. Note the colour of the lesions and the linear shape of some of them.

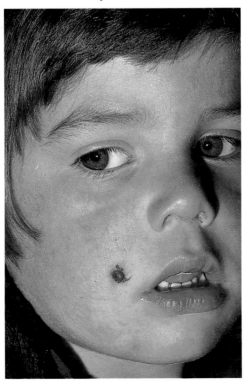

**5.52** Pyogenic granuloma.

**Non-erythematous lesions**
**Warty (papillomatous) surface**
**Papules, plaques and nodules**
**Brown/skin colour**

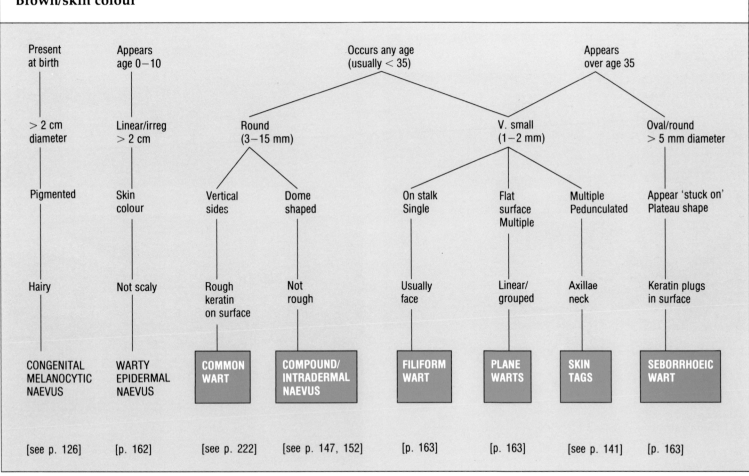

| Present at birth | Appears age 0–10 | Occurs any age (usually < 35) | | | | Appears over age 35 | |
|---|---|---|---|---|---|---|---|

Present at birth → > 2 cm diameter → Pigmented → Hairy → CONGENITAL MELANOCYTIC NAEVUS [see p. 126]

Appears age 0–10 → Linear/irreg > 2 cm → Skin colour → Not scaly → WARTY EPIDERMAL NAEVUS [p. 162]

Occurs any age (usually < 35) → Round (3–15 mm):
- Vertical sides → Rough keratin on surface → COMMON WART [see p. 222]
- Dome shaped → Not rough → COMPOUND/ INTRADERMAL NAEVUS [see p. 147, 152]

V. small (1–2 mm):
- On stalk Single → Usually face → FILIFORM WART [p. 163]
- Flat surface Multiple → Linear/ grouped → PLANE WARTS [p. 163]
- Multiple Pedunculated → Axillae neck → SKIN TAGS [see p. 141]

Appears over age 35 → Oval/round > 5 mm diameter → Appear 'stuck on' Plateau shape → Keratin plugs in surface → SEBORRHOEIC WART [p. 163]

## WARTY EPIDERMAL NAEVUS

An epidermal naevus is a developmental defect where there is overgrowth of the epidermis. Clinically it presents as a brown or skin coloured linear plaque of warty skin, occurring during childhood and remaining fixed in site. It may be quite small (1–2 cm) or occur down the length of a limb or unilaterally around the trunk.

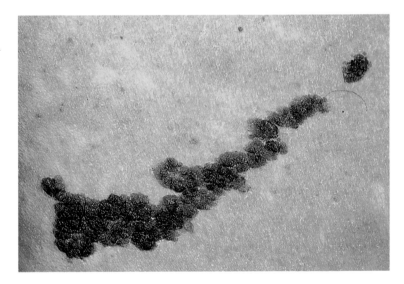

**5.54** Warty epidermal naevus: it has been present since birth.

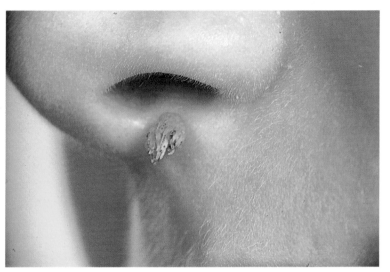

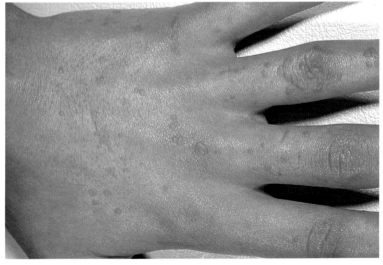

*Right above*
**5.55** Filiform wart.

*Right below*
**5.56** Plane warts.

## FILIFORM WARTS

These are long thin warts on a stalk and are common around the eyelids, nose and beard area.

## PLANE WARTS

These are small flat-topped papules, but unlike the papules of lichen planus they are not shiny. They are not rough to the touch like common warts, but are skin coloured, pink or brown in colour, and may be found in straight lines at sites of trauma (Koebner phenomenon). They occur mainly in children on the dorsum of the hands and on the face.

## SEBORRHOEIC WART (BASAL CELL PAPILLOMA)

These very common lesions have a flat but warty surface, and typically look as if they are 'stuck on' to the skin. Sometimes small keratin cysts can be seen in the surface. Initially they are skin coloured and not very noticeable, but gradually become more prominent and deepen in colour so that their colour varies from light brown to sometimes jet black. They are often multiple but tend to be isolated rather than in a circumscribed group. With increasing age they occur more frequently and increase in number.

Once the diagnosis has been considered, they should not cause any diagnostic confusion. Their appearance late in life, changing colour and increase in elevation are all features that cause alarm to the patient and result in referral for specialist opinion. Occasionally they may become inflamed, particularly if they have been caught in clothing and partly torn off (Fig. 5.51, p. 159). They need to be distinguished from moles, solar keratoses, and occasionally from

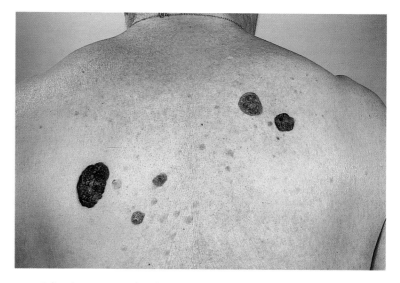

**5.57** Seborrhoeic warts (basal cell papillomas) on the back: variable colour but they all look as if they are 'stuck on' to the surface.

pigmented basal cell carcinomas and malignant melanomas. Moles (melanocytic naevi) are more dome shaped and do not have the 'stuck on' appearance, while solar keratoses are rough to palpation, being felt more easily than seen. A basal cell carcinoma has a more shiny surface and a rolled edge with telangiectasia; a malignant melanoma has an irregular edge, variation in colour and no 'stuck on' appearance.

**Non-erythematous lesions/rash**
**Scaly/horny/keratin/rough surface**
**Papules and plaques**
**1 Multiple/widespread lesions/rash**

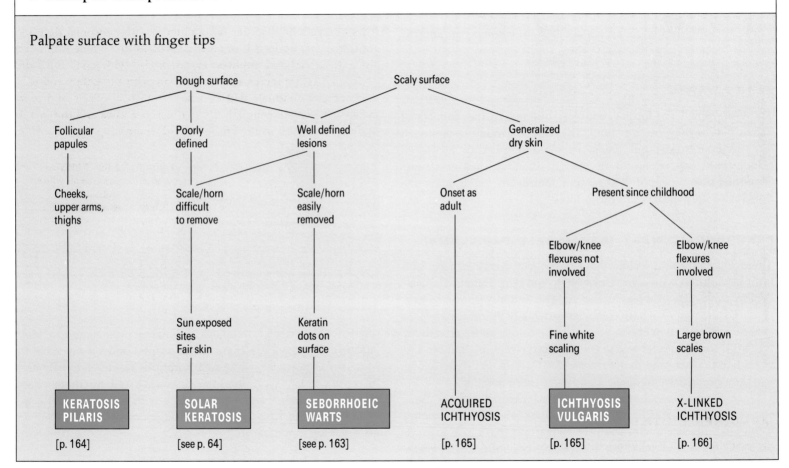

Palpate surface with finger tips

Rough surface

Scaly surface

Follicular papules

Poorly defined

Well defined lesions

Generalized dry skin

Cheeks, upper arms, thighs

Scale/horn difficult to remove

Scale/horn easily removed

Onset as adult

Present since childhood

Elbow/knee flexures not involved

Elbow/knee flexures involved

Sun exposed sites Fair skin

Keratin dots on surface

Fine white scaling

Large brown scales

**KERATOSIS PILARIS**

**SOLAR KERATOSIS**

**SEBORRHOEIC WARTS**

ACQUIRED ICHTHYOSIS

**ICHTHYOSIS VULGARIS**

X-LINKED ICHTHYOSIS

[p. 164]

[see p. 64]

[see p. 163]

[p. 165]

[p. 165]

[p. 166]

## KERATOSIS PILARIS

This is caused by blockage of the hair follicles by horny plugs. It is very common in childhood and adolescence. Skin coloured follicular papules develop on the cheeks and over the upper arms and thighs. Sometimes the papules are red rather than skin coloured. It may be associated with ichthyosis vulgaris or atopic eczema, and is often familial.

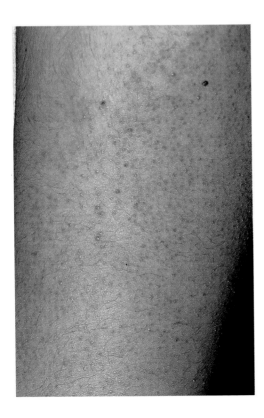

**5.58** Keratosis pilaris of upper arm: tiny follicular papules.

## ICHTHYOSIS VULGARIS

This is a genetic disorder transmitted as an autosomal dominant trait. It is first noticed at or soon after birth: the whole skin except the anti-cubital and popliteal fossae, is dry with small fine white scales. There are increased skin markings on the palms and soles, and some individuals will also have keratosis pilaris and atopic eczema. The main complaint is of the appearance and the itching: it often improves in the sun and with increasing age.

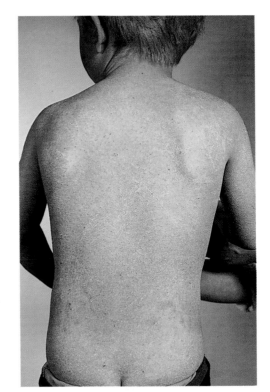

**5.59** Ichthyosis vulgaris: small white scales and excoriations.

## ACQUIRED ICHTHYOSIS

This is similar clinically to ichthyosis vulgaris but occurs later in life. It may be idiopathic or due to an underlying lymphoma.

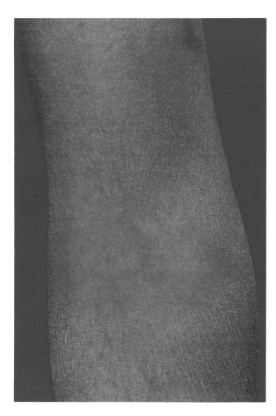

**5.60** Ichthyosis vulgaris sparing the antecubital fossa.

## X-LINKED ICHTHYOSIS

This is transmitted by an X-linked recessive gene, so appears in boys but is transmitted through females. It is much less common than ichthyosis vulgaris from which it is distinguished by the fact that the scales are large and dirty-brown in colour and the flexures are involved. Sunshine does not help and it does not usually improve with age.

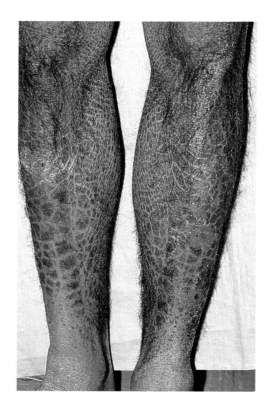

**5.61** X-linked ichthyosis: large brown scales.

**Non-erythematous lesions**
**Scaly/horny/keratin/rough surface**
**Papules, plaques and nodules**
**2 Single/few (1–5) lesions**

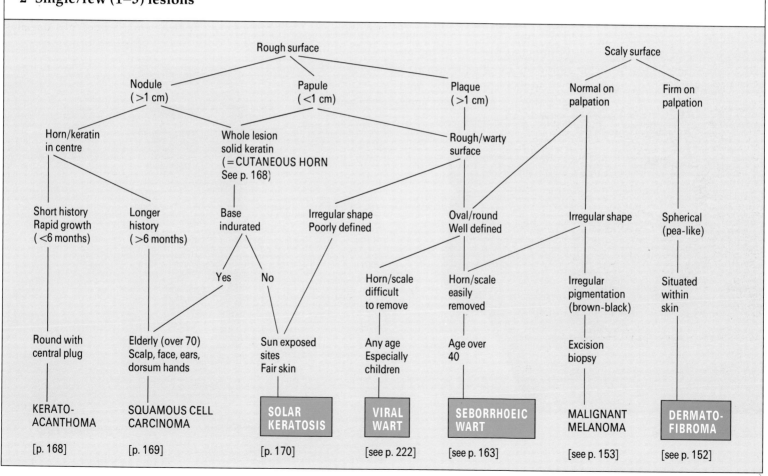

## KERATOACANTHOMA

A rapidly growing benign tumour occurring on sun exposed skin. It enlarges rapidly for about 3 months, remains static and then regresses spontaneously. It should not be present for more than 6 months. It has a typical symmetrical configuration with an erythematous or translucent circumference and a horny volcano-like centre. It may look like a basal cell carcinoma but its fast growth and production of keratin in the centre should distinguish it. A well-differentiated squamous cell carcinoma tends to be more irregular in shape, slower growing and does not regress spontaneously.

## CUTANEOUS HORN

This term is used to describe a horny outgrowth. It is not a diagnosis; it usually overlies a solar keratosis, Bowen's disease, or squamous cell carcinoma. A viral wart may occasionally be confused with a cutaneous horn, but usually has a filiform appearance (see Fig. 5.55, p. 162).

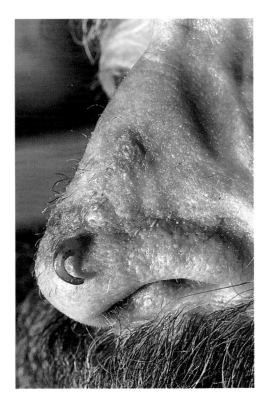

**5.63** Cutaneous horn on nose arising from a solar keratosis.

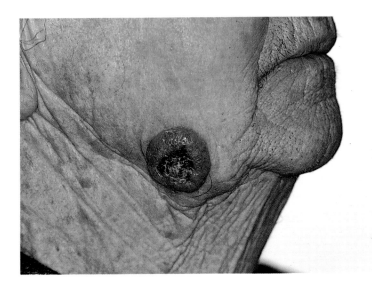

**5.62** Keratoacanthoma.

## SQUAMOUS CELL CARCINOMA

This is a less common neoplasm of the skin than a basal cell carcinoma. The older the patient, the more likely the tumour is to be a squamous cell carcinoma. It may arise from a pre-existing lesion such as a solar keratosis or Bowen's disease. Squamous cell carcinomas occur at sites of maximum sun exposure: on a bald head, the lower lip, cheeks, nose, top of ear lobes and dorsum of the hands. There is usually other evidence of sun damage such as

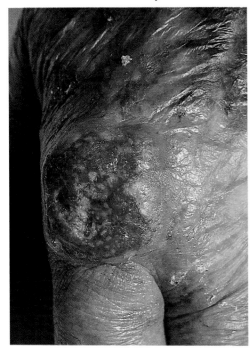

**5.64** Squamous cell carcinoma on the back of the hand.

solar elastosis and solar keratoses. If well differentiated, the tumour may initially be scaly or horny; it is differentiated from a solar keratosis by the induration at its base. Later the tumour may

ulcerate and then be covered by a crust. The edge of the ulcer is craggy and indurated, while the base bleeds easily. It is distinguished from a basal cell carcinoma by its site, the production of keratin and its faster growth (it may grow to 1—2 cm in diameter over a few months). Generally speaking squamous cell carcinomas that arise in sun-damaged skin are less likely to metastasize than squamous cell lesions originating in other parts of the body, e.g. the lung.

Squamous cell carcinomas arising in non-sun-exposed sites can be due to arsenic, previous radiation, chronic scars such as old burn scars, lupus vulgaris (see p. 69) or leg ulcers.

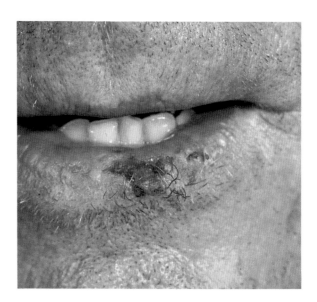

**5.65** Squamous cell carcinoma on the lower lip. Tumours on the lower lip are always sccs until proved otherwise.

## SOLAR KERATOSES

These are typically rough lesions resulting from the production of abnormal keratin in chronically sun-exposed skin. They are commonest on the bald scalp, face and dorsum of the hands, in patients over the age of 50 with fair skin and other evidence of sun damage (see p. 64). Generally they are more easily felt than seen due to the roughness of the abnormal keratin. The surrounding skin may be normal or pink/red. Sometimes scaling is not present and the lesion exists as a fixed red or brown macule.

The diagnosis should not be difficult as nothing else produces such rough scaling on sun-exposed skin in the elderly. Seborrhoeic warts occur in similar patients, but never have the same rough feel to palpation, and are generally seen more easily than felt.

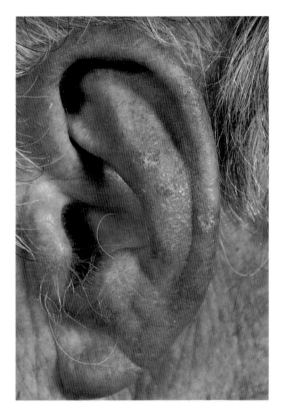

**5.67** Solar keratosis on the ear.

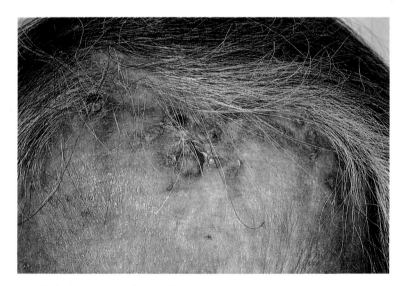

**5.66** Solar keratoses on forehead.

**Non-erythematous/erythematous lesions**
**Crusted, ulcerated or bleeding surface**
**Papules, plaques and nodules**
**1  Single/few (1–5) lesions, fixed site**     **(Multiple lesions ( > 5)/rash, variable in site and time—see chronic erythematous rash p. 122)**

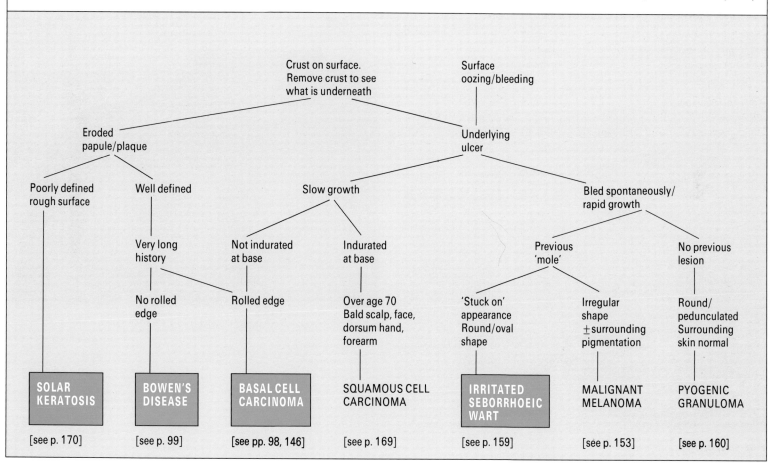

| | | | | | | |
|---|---|---|---|---|---|---|
| SOLAR KERATOSIS | BOWEN'S DISEASE | BASAL CELL CARCINOMA | SQUAMOUS CELL CARCINOMA | IRRITATED SEBORRHOEIC WART | MALIGNANT MELANOMA | PYOGENIC GRANULOMA |
| [see p. 170] | [see p. 99] | [see pp. 98, 146] | [see p. 169] | [see p. 159] | [see p. 153] | [see p. 160] |

**Non-erythematous lesions**
**Hairy surface**
**Patches, papules and plaques**
**Brown colour**

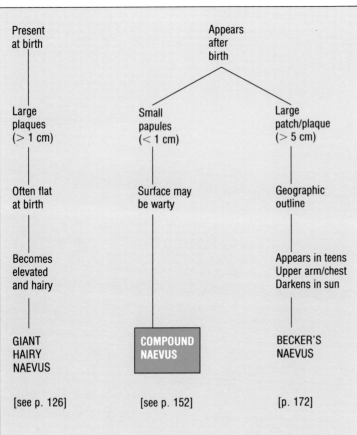

Present at birth → Large plaques (> 1 cm) → Often flat at birth → Becomes elevated and hairy → GIANT HAIRY NAEVUS [see p. 126]

Appears after birth → Small papules (< 1 cm) → Surface may be warty → **COMPOUND NAEVUS** [see p. 152]

Appears after birth → Large patch/plaque (> 5 cm) → Geographic outline → Appears in teens / Upper arm/chest / Darkens in sun → BECKER'S NAEVUS [p. 172]

## BECKER'S NAEVUS

This is an irregular shaped patch of pigmentation associated with increased hairs. It initially develops in the mid–late teens but then persists for life. It is often first noticed after sun exposure. It most commonly occurs over the shoulder region but can occur anywhere.

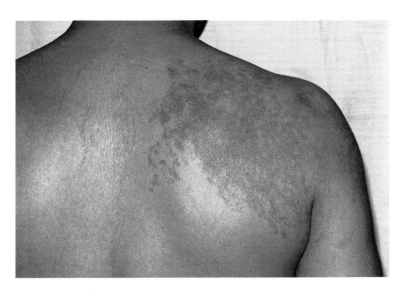

**5.68** Becker's naevus over right shoulder.

# Chapter 6
# Rashes and Lesions in the Flexures: axillae, groins, natal cleft

**Flexures**
**Erythematous lesions/rash**
**Plaques**

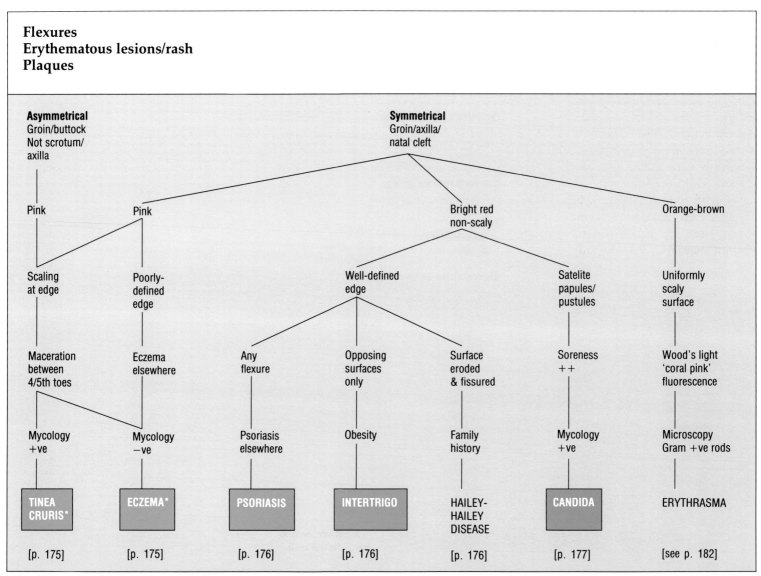

**Asymmetrical**
Groin/buttock
Not scrotum/
axilla

**Symmetrical**
Groin/axilla/
natal cleft

Pink — Scaling at edge — Maceration between 4/5th toes — Mycology +ve — **TINEA CRURIS\*** [p. 175]

Pink — Poorly-defined edge — Eczema elsewhere — Mycology −ve — **ECZEMA\*** [p. 175]

Bright red non-scaly

Well-defined edge — Any flexure — Psoriasis elsewhere — **PSORIASIS** [p. 176]

Well-defined edge — Opposing surfaces only — Obesity — **INTERTRIGO** [p. 176]

Well-defined edge — Surface eroded & fissured — Family history — HAILEY-HAILEY DISEASE [p. 176]

Satelite papules/pustules — Soreness ++ — Mycology +ve — **CANDIDA** [p. 177]

Orange-brown — Uniformly scaly surface — Wood's light 'coral pink' fluorescence — Microscopy Gram +ve rods — ERYTHRASMA [see p. 182]

\* Consider PUBIC LICE if itching/no rash in pubic area (p. 176)

## TINEA CRURIS

Dermatophyte fungal infections in the flexures only occur in the groins and do not involve the axillae, and only the natal cleft and buttocks by direct spread from the groin. The organisms causing it are the same as those causing tinea pedis, i.e. *Trichophyton mentagrophytes*, *Trichophyton rubrum* or *Epidermophyton floccosum*. Infection is nearly always from the patient's own feet and men are affected more often than women.

The rash starts in the fold of the groin and gradually spreads outwards and down the thigh. The leading edge is scaly unless treated with topical steroids when the whole area may become red. The rash is usually asymmetrical, one side being more involved than the other, and the scrotum is often spared. The infection may spread backwards to involve the natal cleft and buttocks.

In practice eczema and tinea involving the groin may be difficult to differentiate, especially if partially treated. Mycological examination is therefore necessary in all groin rashes to establish whether fungus is present (see p. 9).

## FLEXURAL ECZEMA

Eczema in the flexures consists of poorly defined symmetrical pink patches or plaques. In the groin the scrotum often is involved. The eczema may be localized to one or more flexures only or be

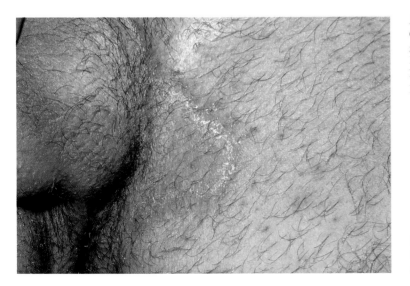

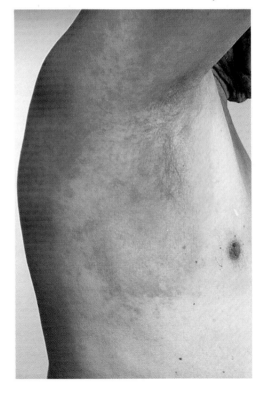

*Left*
**6.1** Tinea cruris: one groin only affected. Notice the scale at the leading edge of the plaque.

*Right*
**6.2** Seborrhoeic eczema in the axilla.

part of seborrhoeic eczema elsewhere. Contact eczema in the axillae may be due to irritants (depilatories, deodorants) or allergens (deodorants, dyes or resins in clothes). Patch testing will distinguish between these.

## PUBIC LICE

If there is itching in the pubic area and not much rash to see, always think of pubic lice. The adults and eggs can be seen firmly attached to the hairs (see p. 270).

## PSORIASIS

Psoriasis of the flexures (any flexure) is distinguished from all other rashes by its bright red colour and well-defined edge. Silvery scaling will not be seen on the moist skin of the flexure, but may be seen at the very edge of the plaque. Often psoriasis is present elsewhere to confirm the diagnosis.

## INTERTRIGO

The word comes from the latin verb *intertrerere* meaning to rub together. In practice intertrigo means painful red skin due to two surfaces rubbing together. It occurs in the summer months in the flexures of individuals who are too fat. It can be distinguished from psoriasis since non-flexural sites are never involved.

## HAILEY-HAILEY DISEASE (CHRONIC BENIGN FAMILIAL PEMPHIGUS)

This rare condition is inherited as an autosomal dominant trait.

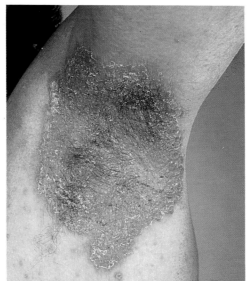

*Far left*
**6.3** Psoriasis of the pubic area.

*Left*
**6.4** Hailey-Hailey disease.

The patient complains of soreness in any of the flexures, and on examination the surface is finely fissured. As in pemphigus there is an abnormality of cohesion of epidermal cells.

## CANDIDIASIS

Candida usually affects patients at the extremes of life, babies and old people, but may also affect adults who are obese or diabetic. It can affect all the flexures (axillae, groins, submammary area, toe webs) and is usually symmetrical. The rash is bright red, and the key feature is that outlying papules or pustules occur away from the main rash. In addition the skin is sore rather than itchy, a feature that may help distinguish it from psoriasis or tinea cruris. Scrapings taken from the edge of the lesions can be examined under the microscope for spores and hyphae (Fig. 1.3, p. 10), or cultured to prove the diagnosis.

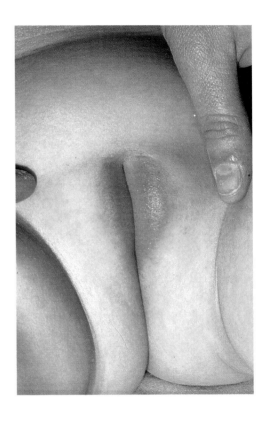

*Right*
**6.6** Candida of vulva: bright red colour, sore rather than itchy.

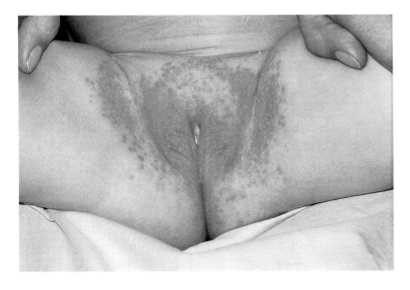

*Left*
**6.5** Candida: note symmetry and outlying papules and pustules.

Flexures—under nappy
Erythematous lesions/rash
Plaques, papules, (pustules), erosions

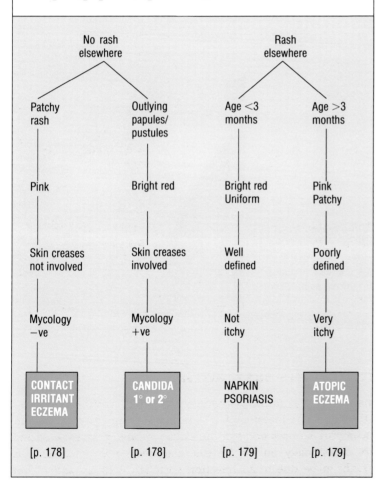

| No rash elsewhere | | Rash elsewhere | |
| --- | --- | --- | --- |
| Patchy rash | Outlying papules/ pustules | Age <3 months | Age >3 months |
| Pink | Bright red | Bright red Uniform | Pink Patchy |
| Skin creases not involved | Skin creases involved | Well defined | Poorly defined |
| Mycology −ve | Mycology +ve | Not itchy | Very itchy |
| **CONTACT IRRITANT ECZEMA** | **CANDIDA 1° or 2°** | NAPKIN PSORIASIS | **ATOPIC ECZEMA** |
| [p. 178] | [p. 178] | [p. 179] | [p. 179] |

## CONTACT IRRITANT ECZEMA (NAPPY RASH)

This is the common type of nappy rash and is an irritant reaction to urine and faeces held next to the skin under occlusion. Bacteria in the faeces split urea in the urine into ammonia which is strongly irritant to the skin. Clinically the rash is patchy and tends to involve the convex skin in contact with the nappy (buttocks, genitalia, thighs) rather than the skin in the folds. In mild cases there is just erythema, but when severe, erosions or even ulcers can develop. The affected area is sore and cleaning or bathing the area produces much discomfort.

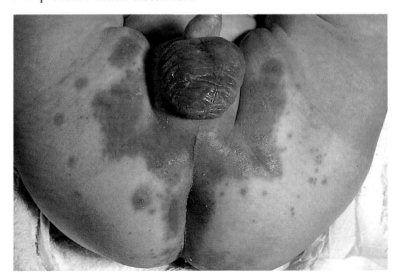

6.7 Nappy rash.

## CANDIDIASIS

Infection of the napkin area with candida can occur as a primary event or secondary to an irritant dermatitis (see p. 177).

## NAPKIN PSORIASIS (INFANTILE SEBORRHOEIC ECZEMA)

Infants under 3 months of age may develop an eruption that looks like psoriasis starting in the nappy area but later spreading to involve the trunk and face. In the nappy area involvement extends into the flexures (unlike ordinary nappy rash); there is no itching and the infant remains unaffected by the rash. The relationship with either psoriasis or seborrhoeic eczema is not known.

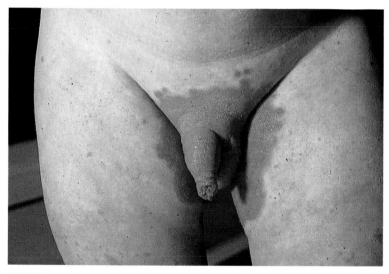

**6.8** Napkin psoriasis.

## ATOPIC ECZEMA

Atopic eczema usually spares the napkin area, but it can occur there too. It occurs after 3 months of age and is very itchy. The rash is eczematous (patchy, pink and ill defined), and is associated with atopic eczema elsewhere, often on the face and scalp (see p. 103).

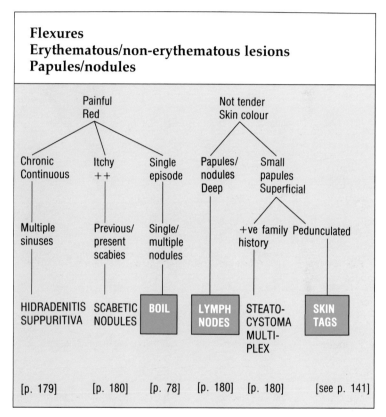

## HIDRADENITIS SUPPURITIVA

This is a disease of the apocrine sweat glands which is localized to the axillae, perineum and areolae. Tender papules, nodules and discharging sinuses occur in the axillae, groins, perineal area and very occasionally on the breasts, and heal to leave scars. It is thought to be due to an infection with *Streptococcus milleri*, but does not always respond to antibiotics.

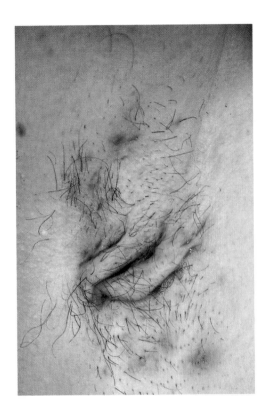

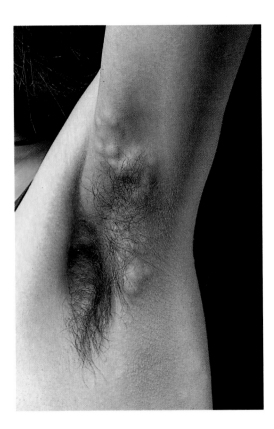

*Far left*
**6.9** Hidradenitis sup-
puritiva in the axilla.

*Left*
**6.10** Steatocystoma
multiplex.

## SCABETIC NODULES

An uncommon sequel to an episode of scabies is persistent, erythematous, itchy papules around the axillae (see p. 116).

## LYMPH NODES

Lymph node enlargement may be reactive to a local infection, or due to malignancy, either a lymphoma or a secondary carcinoma.

## STEATOCYSTOMA MULTIPLEX

This is a rare genetically-determined condition in which multiple small skin-coloured or white papules occur in the flexures or on the trunk of young adults.

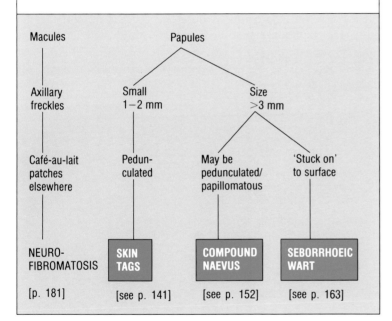

**Flexures**
**Non-erythematous lesions**
**Macules/papules**
**Brown colour**

Macules                          Papules

Axillary              Small                    Size
freckles              1–2 mm                   >3 mm

Café-au-lait          Pedun-       May be           'Stuck on'
patches               culated      pedunculated/    to surface
elsewhere                          papillomatous

NEURO-           **SKIN**      **COMPOUND**    **SEBORRHOEIC**
FIBROMATOSIS     **TAGS**      **NAEVUS**      **WART**

[p. 181]         [see p. 141]  [see p. 152]    [see p. 163]

## NEUROFIBROMATOSIS

'Axillary freckles' or light brown macules are pathognomic of neurofibromatosis. In children this sign may pre-date the development of the neurofibromas, but there will be café-au-lait patches elsewhere on the trunk (see p. 128).

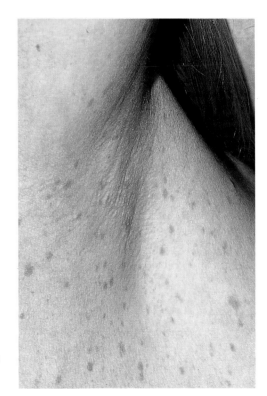

**6.11** Axillary freckling in a patient with neurofibromatosis.

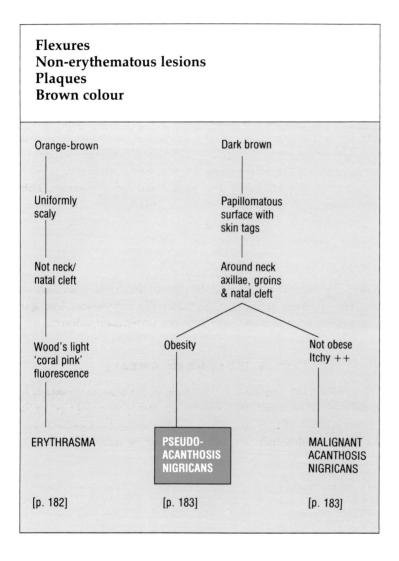

**Flexures**
**Non-erythematous lesions**
**Plaques**
**Brown colour**

Orange-brown

Uniformly
scaly

Not neck/
natal cleft

Wood's light
'coral pink'
fluorescence

ERYTHRASMA

[p. 182]

Dark brown

Papillomatous
surface with
skin tags

Around neck
axillae, groins
& natal cleft

Obesity

**PSEUDO-
ACANTHOSIS
NIGRICANS**

[p. 183]

Not obese
Itchy ++

MALIGNANT
ACANTHOSIS
NIGRICANS

[p. 183]

## ERYTHRASMA

Erythrasma is a bacterial infection (*Propionibacterium minutissimum*) of the flexures. Symmetrical orangy-brown scaly plaques spread out from the folds. Usually all flexures are involved; axillae, groins, submammary areas and toe clefts. It may be confused with tinea cruris, but the colour is different, there is no scaly leading edge, the axillae are involved and mycology will be negative. A Gram stain on the scales will reveal Gram positive diphtheroids, and Wood's light (UVA) examination reveals a coral pink fluorescence.

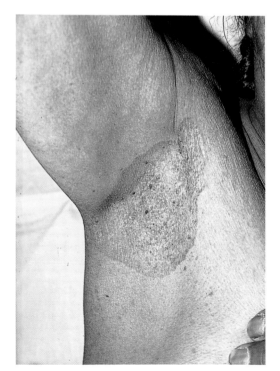

**6.12** Erythrasma.

## ACANTHOSIS NIGRICANS

This is a rare condition but important, because if it occurs over the age of 40 you should look for an underlying malignancy. The skin of the neck and flexures becomes dark brown, dry, and thickened with a papillomatous velvety surface. The skin markings may be accentuated and small skin tags appear. In the malignant form the skin changes are often associated with marked itching.

Pseudo-acanthosis nigricans looks the same but occurs in those who are obese, and will disappear if the patient loses weight.

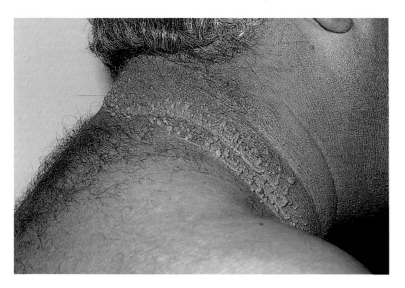

6.13 Acanthosis nigricans.

## ABNORMALITIES OF SWEATING

### AXILLARY HYPERHIDROSIS

Eccrine sweat glands are distributed all over the body surface. They consist of tight secretory coils situated deep in the dermis, linked to the surface by straight ducts opening directly onto the surface. An isotonic secretion is produced in the coil, and this may be modified as it passes up the duct. Secretion of sweat is stimulated by the sympathetic nerves via a cholinergic neuro-transmitter. The stimulus for sweat glands in the axillae, palms and soles is emotional rather than thermoregulatory. Axillary hyperhidrosis is embarrassing as it may ruin the clothes.

### BROMHIDROSIS

Odour of the skin is probably due to bacterial breakdown of axillary apocrine secretions. Occasionally substances like garlic secreted in eccrine sweat can produce unpleasant odours.

### CHROMHIDROSIS (COLOURED SWEAT)

Apocrine sweat may be coloured yellow, blue or green when it is secreted. More commonly colourless apocrine sweat is broken down to different colours by bacteria on the skin surface or on axillary or pubic hair. The main problem is staining of clothing.

## TRICHOMYCOSIS AXILLARIS

This is a very common superficial infection of axillary or pubic hairs with a variety of propionibacteria. White or coloured concretions are fixed to the hair. Most people do not notice this but occasionally some complain of it.

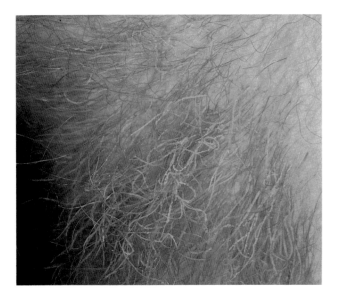

**6.14** Trichomycosis axillaris (Courtesy of Dr M. E. Kesseler).

# Chapter 7
# Rashes and Lesions affecting principally the Lower Legs

**Lower legs**
**Acute erythematous lesions/rash**
**Normal/exudative surface**
**Patches, papules, plaques, blisters**

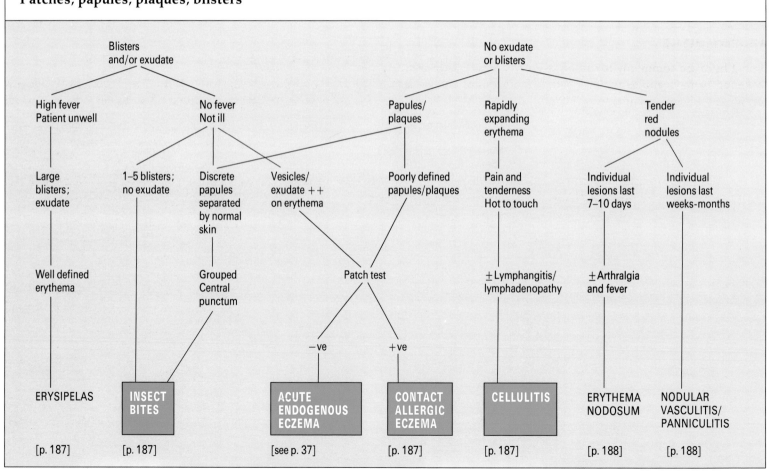

## ERYSIPELAS

This is an infection of the upper half of the dermis with a group A beta haemolytic streptococcus. A well-defined red swollen area with central blistering occurs with no obvious portal of entry for the bacteria (see p. 44).

## INSECT BITES

Insect bites are commonly found on the lower legs. Discrete skin-coloured or red papules with a central punctum are typical; less commonly blisters occur (see p. 119).

## CONTACT ALLERGIC ECZEMA

Contact allergic eczema on the lower legs is usually due to medicaments applied for the treatment of venous eczema or ulcers. The common sensitizers are various antibiotics (neomycin, soframycin, fucidin), lanolin, parabens (a preservative in creams and paste bandages), and occasionally the rubber in elastic support bandages.

## CELLULITIS

This is an infection of the lower half of the dermis by a group A, C or G beta haemolytic streptococcus. There is usually an obvious

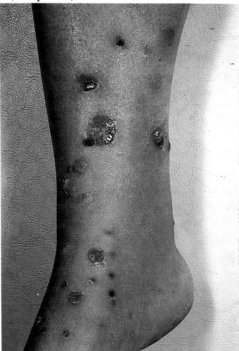

7.1 Insect bites on the lower leg.

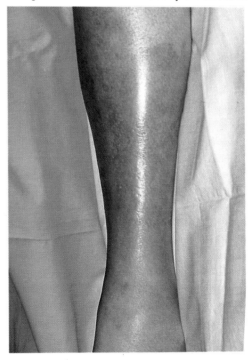

7.2 Cellulitis.

portal of entry for the organism, such as a leg ulcer, tinea between the toes or eczema on the feet or legs. It looks like erysipelas except that the area of erythema is less well defined, and there is associated lymphangitis and lymphadenopathy. There are no blisters and the patient is less unwell.

## ERYTHEMA NODOSUM

Tender red nodules appear on the front of the shins mainly in young women. Individual lesions are 1–10 cm in diameter, initially bright red in colour, but fading through the colour changes of a bruise over 7–10 days. Lesions come in crops for 3–6 weeks. There may be associated general malaise, fever and arthropathy. It may be due to a streptococcal throat infection, sarcoidosis, drugs (particularly sulphonamides and the contraceptive pill), tuberculosis, and numerous other bacterial, rickettsial or viral infections. Sometimes no cause can be found.

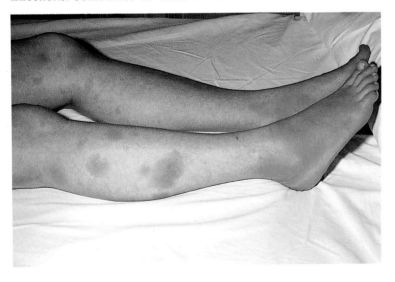

## NODULAR VASCULITIS/PANNICULITIS

One or several tender red nodules on the lower legs which persist for weeks or months are due to nodular vasculitis or nodular panniculitis. They can only be distinguished by biopsy, and a referral to a specialist is necessary to sort out the cause.

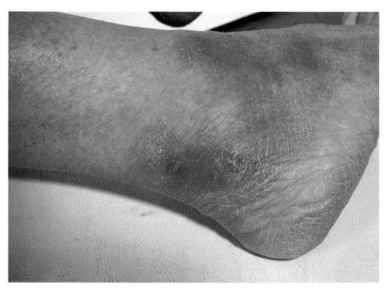

**7.4** Nodular vasculitis.

**7.3** Erythema nodosum.

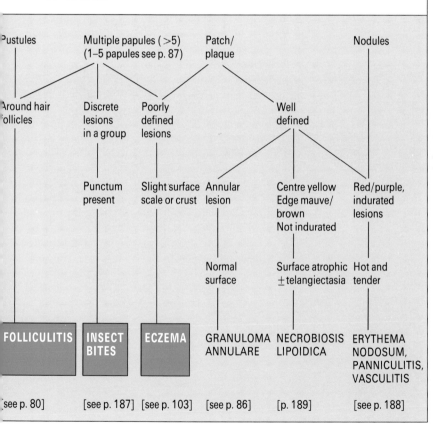

**Lower legs**
**Chronic erythematous lesions/rash**
**Surface normal**

Pustules

Multiple papules (>5)
(1–5 papules see p. 87)

Patch/
plaque

Nodules

Around hair
follicles

Discrete
lesions
in a group

Poorly
defined
lesions

Well
defined

Punctum
present

Slight surface
scale or crust

Annular
lesion

Centre yellow
Edge mauve/
brown
Not indurated

Red/purple,
indurated
lesions

Normal
surface

Surface atrophic
±telangiectasia

Hot and
tender

| FOLLICULITIS | INSECT BITES | ECZEMA | GRANULOMA ANNULARE | NECROBIOSIS LIPOIDICA | ERYTHEMA NODOSUM, PANNICULITIS, VASCULITIS |
|---|---|---|---|---|---|
| [see p. 80] | [see p. 187] | [see p. 103] | [see p. 86] | [p. 189] | [see p. 188] |

## NECROBIOSIS LIPOIDICA

This condition is confined to the front of the shins. A well-defined round or oval plaque with a raised mauve or brown edge and a yellow atrophic centre in which telangiectasia is obvious is characteristic. Occasionally the atrophic area may ulcerate. Seventy percent of patients with this condition are diabetic but there seems to be no relationship between the appearance or spread of the skin disease and control of the diabetes.

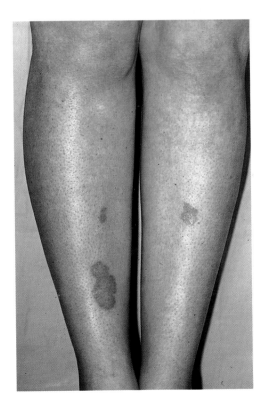

**7.5** Necrobiosis lipoidica.

**Lower leg**
**Chronic erythematous rash/lesions**
**Scaly surface**
**Papules and plaques**

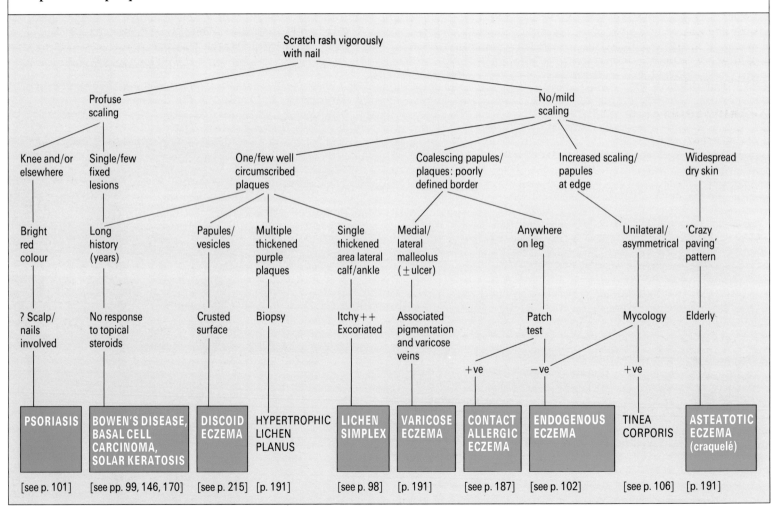

Scratch rash vigorously with nail

Profuse scaling → Knee and/or elsewhere → Bright red colour → ? Scalp/nails involved → **PSORIASIS** [see p. 101]

Profuse scaling → Single/few fixed lesions → Long history (years) → No response to topical steroids → **BOWEN'S DISEASE, BASAL CELL CARCINOMA, SOLAR KERATOSIS** [see pp. 99, 146, 170]

One/few well circumscribed plaques → Papules/vesicles → Crusted surface → **DISCOID ECZEMA** [see p. 215]

One/few well circumscribed plaques → Multiple thickened purple plaques → Biopsy → **HYPERTROPHIC LICHEN PLANUS** [p. 191]

No/mild scaling → One/few well circumscribed plaques → Single thickened area lateral calf/ankle → Itchy++ Excoriated → **LICHEN SIMPLEX** [see p. 98]

Coalescing papules/plaques: poorly defined border → Medial/lateral malleolus (±ulcer) → Associated pigmentation and varicose veins → **VARICOSE ECZEMA** [p. 191]

Coalescing papules/plaques: poorly defined border → Anywhere on leg → Patch test → +ve → **CONTACT ALLERGIC ECZEMA** [see p. 187]

Patch test → −ve → **ENDOGENOUS ECZEMA** [see p. 102]

Increased scaling/papules at edge → Unilateral/asymmetrical → Mycology → +ve → **TINEA CORPORIS** [see p. 106]

No/mild scaling → Widespread dry skin → 'Crazy paving' pattern → Elderly → **ASTEATOTIC ECZEMA (craquelé)** [p. 191]

## HYPERTROPHIC LICHEN PLANUS

Multiple itchy, thickened, pink-purple or violaceous plaques on the lower legs may be due to lichen planus. The surface is slightly scaly and warty and there may be hyperpigmentation. The presence of typical lichen planus elsewhere will suggest the diagnosis, but an isolated plaque needs to be distinguished from lichen simplex by skin biopsy.

## VARICOSE/STASIS ECZEMA

Eczema may occur in patients who have lost the valves in their deep and/or perforating veins. It is distinguished from other types of eczema by being confined to the lower legs in a patient with other signs of venous disease (see p. 193).

## ASTEATOTIC ECZEMA (ECZEMA CRAQUELÉ)

This is due to drying out of the skin especially in the elderly. It occurs in the winter or when patients are hospitalized and made to bathe more frequently than they are used to. The skin is dry and scaly with irregular erythematous fissures like 'crazy paving'. The associated itching causes the patient to complain.

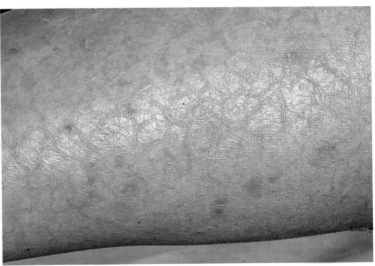

**7.7** Asteototic eczema on the lower leg.

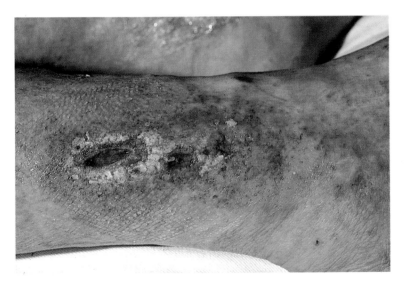

**7.6** Varicose eczema around an ulcer on the lateral aspect of the lower leg.

**Lower legs**
**Chronic erythematous lesions/rash**
**Crusted/exudative surface**
**Papules, plaques and nodules**

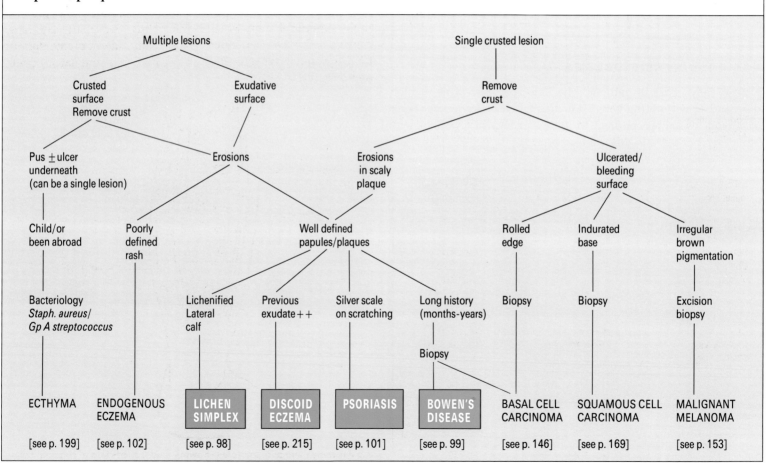

Multiple lesions

Single crusted lesion

Crusted surface
Remove crust

Exudative surface

Remove crust

Pus ±ulcer underneath (can be a single lesion)

Erosions

Erosions in scaly plaque

Ulcerated/ bleeding surface

Child/or been abroad

Poorly defined rash

Well defined papules/plaques

Rolled edge

Indurated base

Irregular brown pigmentation

Bacteriology
*Staph. aureus/ Gp A streptococcus*

Lichenified Lateral calf

Previous exudate++

Silver scale on scratching

Long history (months-years)

Biopsy

Biopsy

Excision biopsy

Biopsy

| ECTHYMA | ENDOGENOUS ECZEMA | **LICHEN SIMPLEX** | **DISCOID ECZEMA** | **PSORIASIS** | **BOWEN'S DISEASE** | BASAL CELL CARCINOMA | SQUAMOUS CELL CARCINOMA | MALIGNANT MELANOMA |
|---|---|---|---|---|---|---|---|---|
| [see p. 199] | [see p. 102] | [see p. 98] | [see p. 215] | [see p. 101] | [see p. 99] | [see p. 146] | [see p. 169] | [see p. 153] |

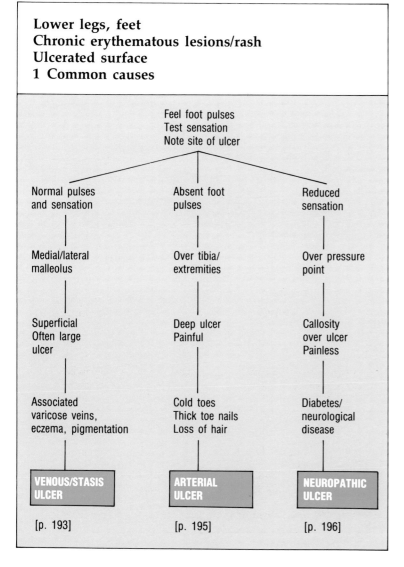

**Lower legs, feet**
**Chronic erythematous lesions/rash**
**Ulcerated surface**
**1 Common causes**

Feel foot pulses
Test sensation
Note site of ulcer

| Normal pulses and sensation | Absent foot pulses | Reduced sensation |
|---|---|---|
| Medial/lateral malleolus | Over tibia/ extremities | Over pressure point |
| Superficial Often large ulcer | Deep ulcer Painful | Callosity over ulcer Painless |
| Associated varicose veins, eczema, pigmentation | Cold toes Thick toe nails Loss of hair | Diabetes/ neurological disease |
| VENOUS/STASIS ULCER | ARTERIAL ULCER | NEUROPATHIC ULCER |
| [p. 193] | [p. 195] | [p. 196] |

## VENOUS ULCERS

Ulceration of the lower leg is most commonly due to venous disease. The first stage is loss of the valves in the deep or perforating veins following a deep vein thrombosis. With the valves gone, contraction of the calf muscles produces enormous pressure in the superficial veins which is transmitted back to the capillaries causing oedema, purpura (leading to haemosiderin pigmentation), dilated venules (venous flare), varicose veins and later eczema and ulceration.

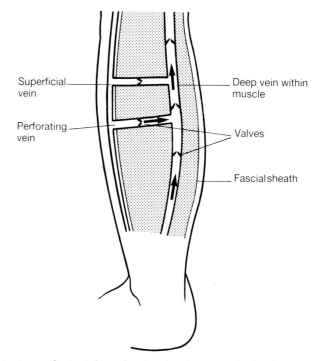

Superficial vein
Perforating vein
Deep vein within muscle
Valves
Fascial sheath

**7.8** Anatomy of veins in lower leg showing deep, superficial and communicating veins with one way valves.

Venous ulcers occur on the lower third of the leg over either the medial or lateral malleolus. They are large, superficial and painless. There will be other evidence of venous disease such as oedema, varicose veins, venous flare, pigmentation (orangey brown due to haemosiderin or dark brown due to melanin), eczema, atrophie blanche (white scars with telangiectasis on the surface), and fibrosis around the ankle.

Complications of venous ulceration are relatively rare, and include cellulitis, haemorrhage, soft tissue calcification and

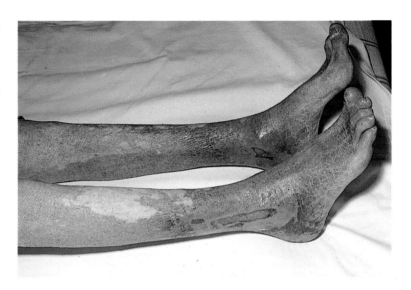

*Left*
**7.9** Venous ulcer: note surrounding eczema and pigmentation.

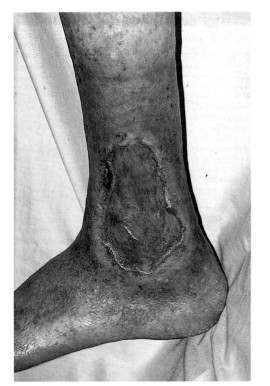

*Right above*
**7.10** Venous ulcer: surrounding hyper-pigmentation due to melanin.

*Right below*
**7.11** Venous flare along the medial border of the foot in a patient with venous ulcers.

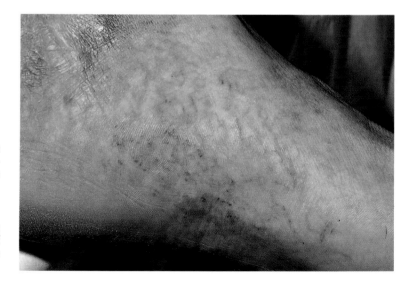

malignant change. Infection of the ulcer itself is of little consequence and mixed organisms are often present. Taking swabs for bacteriology should be discouraged as this tempts the physician to treat with potentially sensitizing topical antibiotics. Cellulitis should be treated promptly, but this diagnosis is made on clinical grounds (see p. 187).

will confirm the diagnosis. Other signs to look for are cold feet, blotchy erythema of the feet, loss of hair, and thickened atrophic toenails. Untreated, gangrene will eventually follow. The patient may have evidence of more widespread arterial disease such as a past history of coronary thrombosis or stroke.

Venous ulcers may be complicated by arterial insufficiency, and this is suggested by pain and poor healing with compression bandages.

**7.12** Atrophie blanche: white scar with telangiectasia within, occuring in a patient with previous venous ulceration.

### ARTERIAL ULCERS

Arterial ulcers are due to a reduction in arterial blood supply to the lower limb and are usually due to atherosclerosis. They are typically painful, punched out and relatively deep (sometimes revealing the underlying tendons). They occur where the arterial supply is poorest: the tips of the toes, the dorsum of the foot, the heel and the middle of the shin. The absence of peripheral pulses

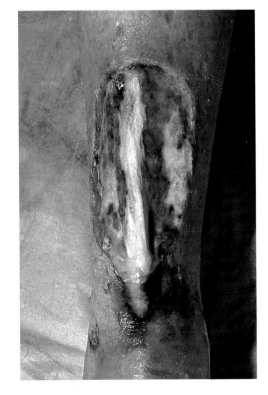

**7.13** Arterial ulcer on the front of the shin. The ulcer is deep with flexor tendon showing.

## NEUROPATHIC ULCERS

These ulcers result from trauma to anaesthetic feet, so occur over bony prominences, particularly the first metatarsophalangeal joint, the metatarsal heads, the heel, or at any site of injury. Classically they are deep, painless, and often covered with thick callous.

The diagnosis is confirmed by finding sensory loss and some associated disorder that has caused it, e.g. diabetes, leprosy, paraplegia, peripheral nerve injury, polyneuropathy, syringomyelia etc.

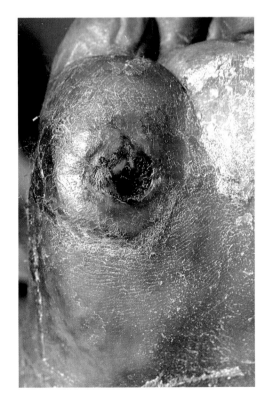

**7.14** Neuropathic ulcer: note hyperkeratosis around ulcer.

**Lower legs/feet**
**Chronic erythematous lesions/rash**
**Ulcerated surface** *Consider if pulses normal
**2 Uncommon causes*** sensation normal
no evidence of venous stasis

In Negro consider SICKLE CELL DISEASE (p. 198)
Recent travel to tropics consider TROPICAL ULCERS (p. 198)
ECTHYMA (p. 199)
LEISHMANIASIS (p. 200)

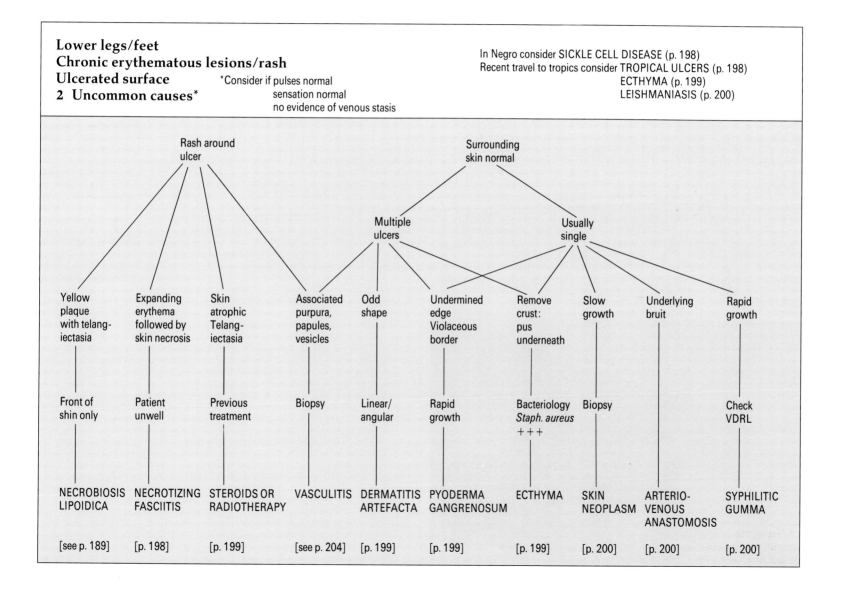

| | | | | | | | | | |
|---|---|---|---|---|---|---|---|---|---|
| **Rash around ulcer** | | | | **Surrounding skin normal** | | | | | |
| | | | | Multiple ulcers | | Usually single | | | |
| Yellow plaque with telang-iectasia | Expanding erythema followed by skin necrosis | Skin atrophic Telang-iectasia | Associated purpura, papules, vesicles | Odd shape | Undermined edge Violaceous border | Remove crust: pus underneath | Slow growth | Underlying bruit | Rapid growth |
| Front of shin only | Patient unwell | Previous treatment | Biopsy | Linear/angular | Rapid growth | Bacteriology *Staph. aureus* +++ | Biopsy | | Check VDRL |
| NECROBIOSIS LIPOIDICA | NECROTIZING FASCIITIS | STEROIDS OR RADIOTHERAPY | VASCULITIS | DERMATITIS ARTEFACTA | PYODERMA GANGRENOSUM | ECTHYMA | SKIN NEOPLASM | ARTERIO-VENOUS ANASTOMOSIS | SYPHILITIC GUMMA |
| [see p. 189] | [p. 198] | [p. 199] | [see p. 204] | [p. 199] | [p. 199] | [p. 199] | [p. 200] | [p. 200] | [p. 200] |

## SICKLE CELL ULCERS

Ulceration on the lower legs in patients with homozygous sickle cell disease is due to sickling of the red cells causing anoxia to the skin. Minor trauma may then cause ulceration.

## TROPICAL ULCERS

In hot or humid parts of the world minor trauma to the lower leg may be complicated by infection with bacteria, protozoa or fungi.

## NECROTIZING FASCIITIS

This is an acute fulminant infection of the subcutaneous fat and deep fascia by a group A beta haemolytic streptococcus or *Staphylococcus aureus*. A toxin released from the organism causes thrombosis of the blood vessels in the skin and thence necrosis. Initially it looks like cellulitis or erysipelas but purple areas followed by frank necrosis occur within 2–3 days.

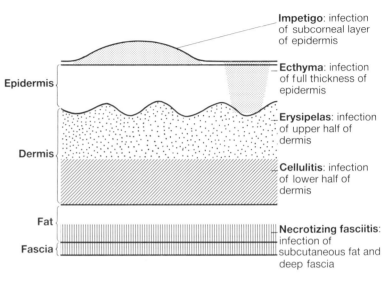

**Impetigo**: infection of subcorneal layer of epidermis

**Ecthyma**: infection of full thickness of epidermis

**Erysipelas**: infection of upper half of dermis

**Cellulitis**: infection of lower half of dermis

**Necrotizing fasciitis**: infection of subcutaneous fat and deep fascia

**7.16** Sites of infections with group A beta-haemolytic streptococcus.

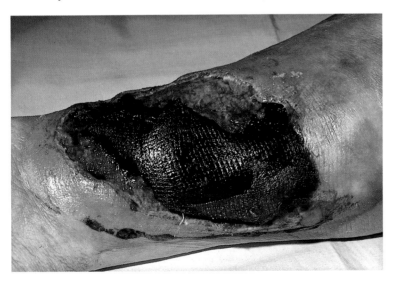

**7.15** Necrotizing fasciitis.

## STEROIDS OR RADIOTHERAPY

Topical or systemic steroids used over long periods, or previous radiotherapy, may result in thinning of dermal collagen and ulceration after minor trauma.

## ECTHYMA

This is an infection of the full thickness of the epidermis by *Staphylococcus aureus* or *Streptococcus pyogenes*. These organisms are usually secondary invaders following injury from an insect bite or other trauma. It presents as a round, punched-out ulcer with a thick crust on top, usually on the leg of a child. It may be seen in adults after travel abroad to hot, humid climates.

## DERMATITIS ARTEFACTA

Any ulcer with straight edges (linear, square or triangular) is artefactual until proven otherwise (see p. 119).

## PYODERMA GANGRENOSUM

A rapidly growing ulcer anywhere on the skin with a violaceous overhanging edge and a yellow, honeycomb-like base suggests the diagnosis of pyoderma gangrenosum. This is associated with ulcerative colitis, Crohn's disease, rheumatoid arthritis or myeloma.

7.17 Ecthyma following an insect bite on a child's leg.

7.18 Pyoderma gangrenosum on the back of a lady with ulcerative colitis.

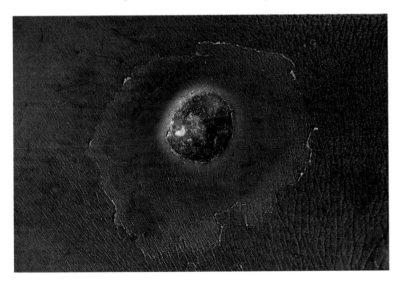

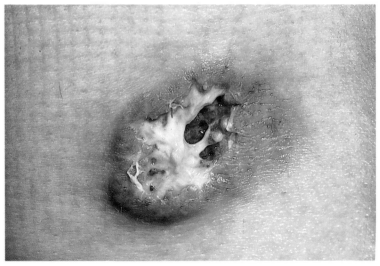

## SKIN NEOPLASM

Malignant melanoma, squamous cell carcinoma and basal cell carcinoma are all rare causes of leg ulcers; chronic non-healing ulcers should therefore be biopsied.

## ARTERIO-VENOUS ANASTOMOSIS

This diagnosis is suggested by a large warm leg with an obvious bruit. It can be a congenital defect or follow a fracture.

## SYPHILITIC GUMMA

A rapidly growing painless ulcer may be a gumma. Always check the VDRL even though gummas are rare today.

## OTHER CAUSES

There are numerous other rare causes of leg ulcers: if in doubt biopsy the ulcer.

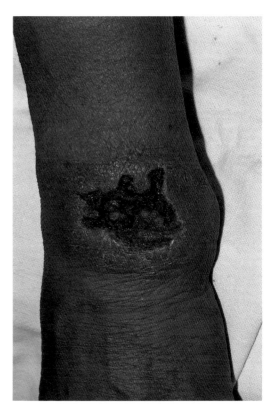

**7.20** Leishmaniasis on the ankle of a 50 year old Iranian woman. This is always worth considering when you see an ulcer in an unusual site in a patient from the Middle East.

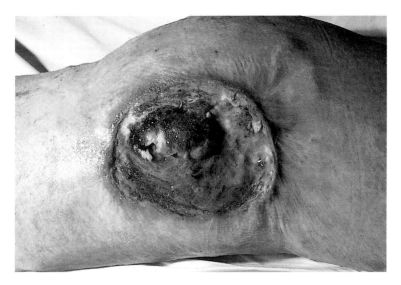

**7.19** Ulcer on medial aspect of right knee: an ulcer at an odd site on the leg should always be biopsied.

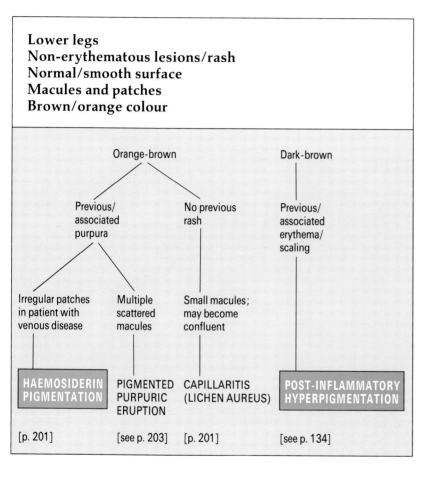

**Lower legs**
**Non-erythematous lesions/rash**
**Normal/smooth surface**
**Macules and patches**
**Brown/orange colour**

Orange-brown

Dark-brown

Previous/
associated
purpura

No previous
rash

Previous/
associated
erythema/
scaling

Irregular patches
in patient with
venous disease

Multiple
scattered
macules

Small macules;
may become
confluent

HAEMOSIDERIN
PIGMENTATION

PIGMENTED
PURPURIC
ERUPTION

CAPILLARITIS
(LICHEN AUREUS)

POST-INFLAMMATORY
HYPERPIGMENTATION

[p. 201]

[see p. 203]

[p. 201]

[see p. 134]

## HAEMOSIDERIN PIGMENTATION

Haemosiderin pigmentation results from purpura from whatever cause (see p. 203). It is orangy-brown in colour. Post-inflammatory hyperpigmentation may be secondary to any inflammatory rash or injury. It commonly follows lichen planus or eczema. It is distinguished from haemosiderin pigmentation by being a darker brown colour.

## CAPILLARITIS

This is a form of vasculitis affecting capillaries. Obvious purpura is not seen, but the remaining haemosiderin deposition is seen as small uniform orange brown macules.

**Lower legs**
**Non-erythematous lesions/rash**
**Surface normal**
**Purpuric − red/purple/orange/brown colour**

Macules/
patches

Lower legs and
other parts
of body

Confined to
lower legs
only

Papules
(palpable
purpura)

Also red
macules/papules/
vesicles/ulcers

Check FBC

Preceding
rash

Venous
disease
present

No other
signs

Biopsy

↓ platelets

Normal

THROMBOCYTOPENIC
PURPURA

CAPILLARITIS/
CORTICOSTEROIDS/
OLD AGE/
OTHER DRUGS

ECZEMA

STASIS
PIGMENT/
PURPURA

PIGMENTED
PURPURIC
ERUPTION

CUTANEOUS
VASCULITIS

[p. 203]     [p. 203]     [see p. 103]     [p. 203]     [p. 203]     [p. 204]

## PURPURA

Purpura is due to leakage of red blood cells from blood vessels into the skin. When compressed with the finger the red colour does not disappear as it would if blood were still inside the blood vessels as in an erythema. The extravasated blood is broken down to haemosiderin causing the colour to change from purple to orange or brown. Purpura may be due to a platelet disorder (*thrombocytopenic purpura*) or a vascular disorder (*non-thrombocytopenic purpura*).

## THROMBOCYTOPENIC PURPURA

If the platelet count falls below $50 \times 10^9$/litre bleeding may occur. In the skin this is seen as tiny purpuric macules and papules (petichiae) and larger patches and plaques (ecchymoses): bleeding may occur elsewhere too. Thrombocytopenia may be due to bone marrow disease (pancytopenia, leukaemia, drug induced marrow failure), systemic infections, splenomegaly or be idiopathic.

## NON-THROMBOCYTOPENIC PURPURA

This can be due to the following:
1 Leaky blood vessels (*capillaritis*). The macules are uniformly small and orangy-brown in colour. It may be idiopathic or due to drugs.
2 Lack of connective tissue support for blood vessels, occuring in old age (*senile purpura*) or after topical or systemic *corticosteroid* therapy. It is seen as easy bruising with large purpuric patches in thin skin which has lost its elasticity (see Figs. 5.19, p. 138).
3 The aftermath of eczema or other *inflammatory conditions* on the lower legs, or as an accompaniment to *venous disease*.
4 *Pigmented purpuric eruption*. Itchy purpura on the lower legs when there is no evidence of eczema is called this; the cause is unknown.

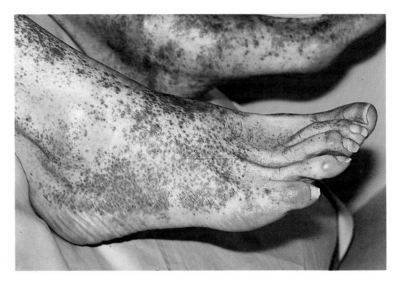

**7.21** Pigmented purpuric eruption.

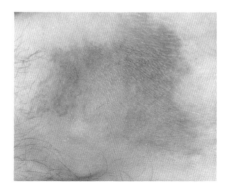

**7.22** Localized pigmented purpuric eruption around ankle, sometimes called lichen aureus because of the golden colour.

## CUTANEOUS VASCULITIS

Vasculitis is usually due to deposition of immune complexes in the small vessels of the skin in patients with a distant focus of infection, a collagen vascular disease, plasma protein abnormality or in those who are taking some drug (e.g. thiazide derivatives, antibiotics or thioureas). The cause may be impossible to identify.

The physical signs are polymorphic with pink or purpuric macules or papules, vesicles and necrotic areas. The skin of the lower legs, feet and buttocks may all be involved. In children it is often associated with painful joints and abdominal pain (*Henoch-Schönlein purpura*).

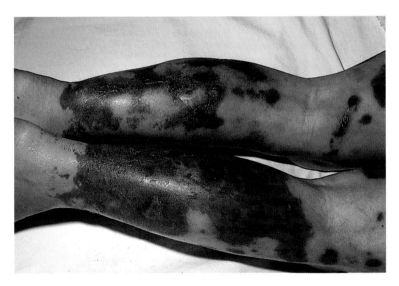

**7.23** Vasculitis due to propyl thiourea.

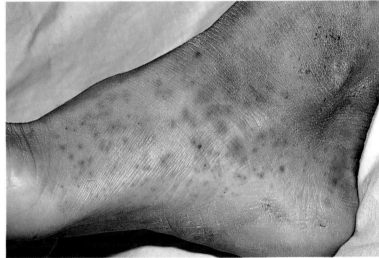

**7.24** Henoch-Schönlein purpura in a boy of 13. Note the polymorphic nature of the lesions: macules, papules, vesicles and crusts.

# Chapter 8
# Hands and Feet (including dorsum of forearms)

## HANDS AND FOREARMS (dorsum)

**Dorsum of fingers/hand/wrist**
**Erythematous rash/lesions**
**1 Single lesion**

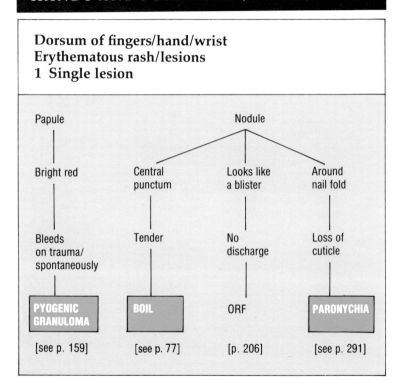

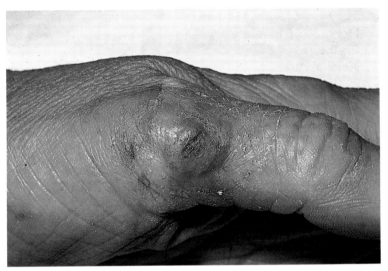

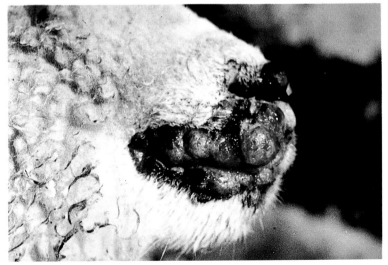

### ORF

Orf is a viral infection of lambs which causes sores around the mouth so that they have difficulty in suckling (Fig. 8.2). It is usually transmitted to humans via a skin cut when bottle feeding affected lambs. It can occasionally be transmitted to housewives and butchers when cleaning a sheep's head. The red, purple or white nodule which develops usually looks like a blister, but no fluid comes out when the nodule is pricked with a needle. It gets better spontaneously after 3—4 weeks.

**Dorsum of hands/forearms**
**Erythematous rash/lesions**
**Normal surface**
**2 Multiple lesions/rash**

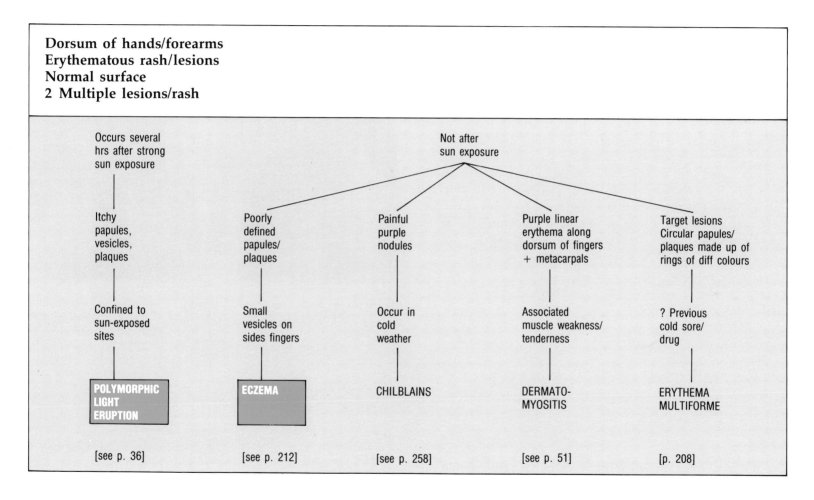

Occurs several
hrs after strong
sun exposure

Not after
sun exposure

Itchy
papules,
vesicles,
plaques

Poorly
defined
papules/
plaques

Painful
purple
nodules

Purple linear
erythema along
dorsum of fingers
+ metacarpals

Target lesions
Circular papules/
plaques made up of
rings of diff colours

Confined to
sun-exposed
sites

Small
vesicles on
sides fingers

Occur in
cold
weather

Associated
muscle weakness/
tenderness

? Previous
cold sore/
drug

**POLYMORPHIC
LIGHT
ERUPTION**

**ECZEMA**

CHILBLAINS

DERMATO-
MYOSITIS

ERYTHEMA
MULTIFORME

[see p. 36]

[see p. 212]

[see p. 258]

[see p. 51]

[p. 208]

*Facing page*

*Above*
**8.1** Orf on a finger.

*Below*
**8.2** Orf on a lamb's mouth. (Courtesy of Coopers Animal Health).

## ERYTHEMA MULTIFORME

This is a distinctive rash occurring 10−14 days after some precipitating cause, e.g. viral infection (especially herpes simplex), bacterial infection (streptococcal sore throat), drug ingestion (sulphonamides, NSAIDS). Multiple small (<1 cm diameter) round papules or blisters made up of rings of different colours (target or iris lesions) occur on the palms, dorsum of hands and forearms, the knees and dorsum of feet. Occasionally they may be widespread and associated with blisters and erosions in the mouth. It may be very itchy but gets better spontaneously after about 10 days. If it follows herpes simplex infections, recurrent episodes can occur.

*Stevens-Johnson syndrome* is erythema multiforme with extensive mucous membrane involvement (see p. 241).

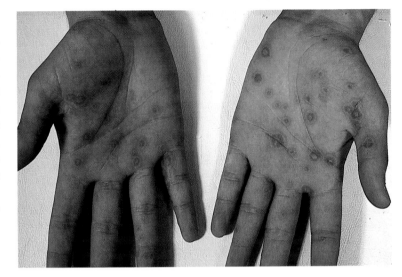

**8.3** Erythema multiforme.

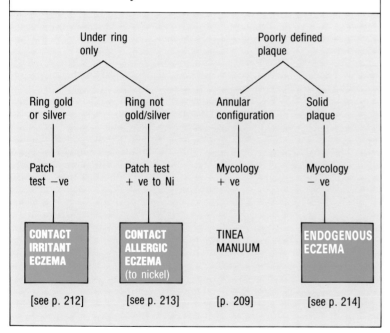

**Dorsum of hand/forearm**
**Erythematous rash/lesions**
**Surface scaly/crust/exudate**
**1 One hand only involved**

Under ring only       Poorly defined plaque

Ring gold or silver    Ring not gold/silver    Annular configuration    Solid plaque

Patch test −ve    Patch test + ve to Ni    Mycology + ve    Mycology − ve

**CONTACT IRRITANT ECZEMA**    **CONTACT ALLERGIC ECZEMA** (to nickel)    TINEA MANUUM    **ENDOGENOUS ECZEMA**

[see p. 212]    [see p. 213]    [p. 209]    [see p. 214]

## TINEA MANUUM

Ringworm infection should be considered in any unilateral red scaly rash, and confirmed or excluded by mycology. The source of the infection is often the patient's own toe webs or nails, so look at the feet as well.

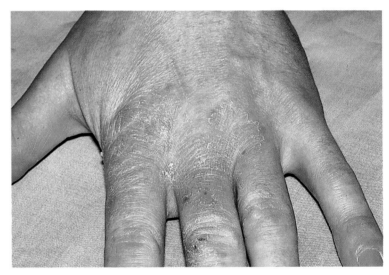

**8.4** Tinea manuum: looks like eczema but on one hand only.

**Dorsum of hand/forearm**
**Erythematous lesions/rash**
**Surface scaly/crust/exudate/horn**
**2  Both hands involved**

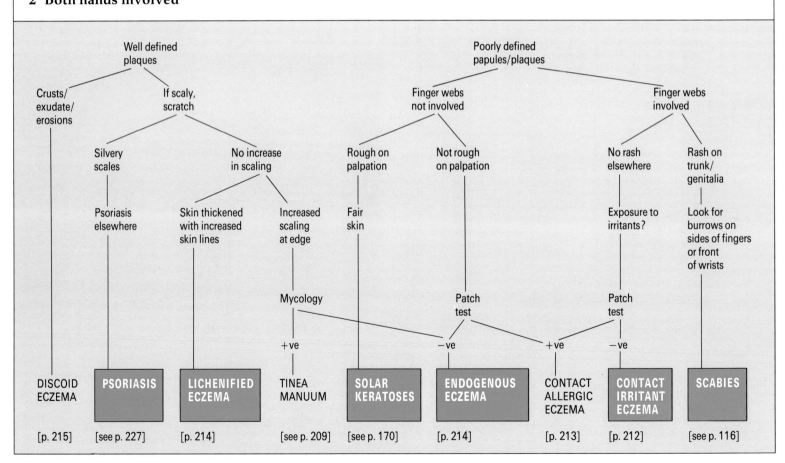

**Palms**
**Erythematous lesions/rash**
**Surface normal/scaly/crust/exudate**
**Papules, plaques, vesicles and pustules**

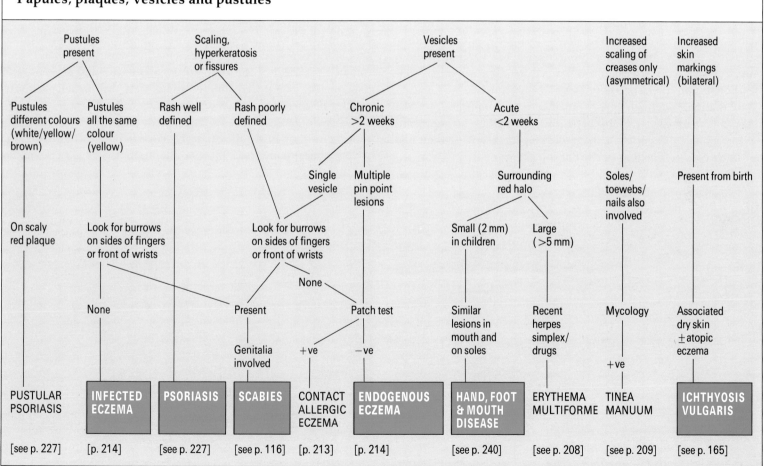

Pustules present

Pustules different colours (white/yellow/brown) — On scaly red plaque — PUSTULAR PSORIASIS [see p. 227]

Pustules all the same colour (yellow) — Look for burrows on sides of fingers or front of wrists — None — INFECTED ECZEMA [p. 214]

Scaling, hyperkeratosis or fissures

Rash well defined — PSORIASIS [see p. 227]

Rash poorly defined — Look for burrows on sides of fingers or front of wrists — Present — Genitalia involved — SCABIES [see p. 116]

None — Patch test

Vesicles present

Chronic >2 weeks

Single vesicle

Multiple pin point lesions

+ve — CONTACT ALLERGIC ECZEMA [p. 213]

−ve — ENDOGENOUS ECZEMA [p. 214]

Acute <2 weeks

Surrounding red halo

Small (2 mm) in children — Similar lesions in mouth and on soles — HAND, FOOT & MOUTH DISEASE [see p. 240]

Large (>5 mm) — Recent herpes simplex/drugs — ERYTHEMA MULTIFORME [see p. 208]

Increased scaling of creases only (asymmetrical)

Soles/toewebs/nails also involved — Mycology +ve — TINEA MANUUM [see p. 209]

Increased skin markings (bilateral)

Present from birth — Associated dry skin ±atopic eczema — ICHTHYOSIS VULGARIS [see p. 165]

## HAND ECZEMA/DERMATITIS

'Eczema' and 'dermatitis' are used interchangeably. Because of the problems of litigation, it is better to call all such rashes eczema unless you are sure that there is an occupational cause.

All types of eczema can occur on the dorsum of the hands. They may be divided into those which are caused by internal factors, *endogenous eczema*, and those caused by external factors, *exogenous eczema.* In practice the cause of the eczema is often multifactorial, with external factors precipitating eczema in a constitutionally predisposed individual.

Occupational dermatitis has medico-legal implications. The assessment of each patient depends on whether he/she could have reasonably expected to have developed eczema if they had not been engaged in that particular job.

### Exogenous eczema

Exogenous eczema may be divided into two types.

### 1. Contact irritant eczema

This is due to weak acids or alkalis (e.g. detergents, shampoos, cleaning materials, cement dust etc) coming into contact with the skin, and occurs in anyone who has enough contact with them. This is the commonest type of eczema to occur on the hands and accounts for most of the time off work due to hand eczema. The rash consists of a poorly defined pink, scaly rash usually without vesicles or crusting, with a dry chapped surface.

In women detergents cause most of the trouble. The rash begins under a ring or in the finger webs where the alkaline detergent particles become trapped. Most young mothers will get eczema on

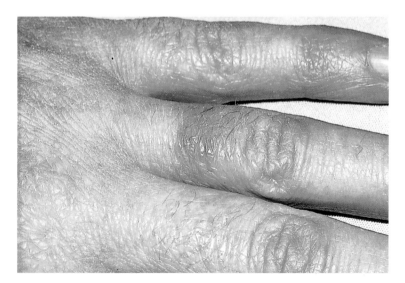

8.5 Contact irritant eczema under a wedding ring (due to detergent trapped there).

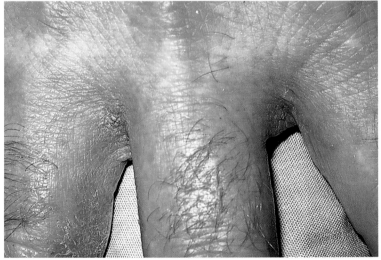

8.6 Contact irritant eczema in the finger webs (due to detergent and inadequate drying between the fingers).

their hands when their children are small. Hairdressers commonly develop irritant eczema when they first begin work due to shampooing. Cooks and nurses are also at risk because of repeated hand washing.

In men contact irritant eczema is mainly on the dorsum of the hands from contact with cement dust or soluble oils used for cooling the moving parts of machinery in the engineering industries.

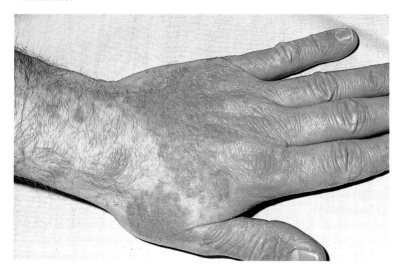

8.7 Contact irritant eczema on the dorsum of the hand due to soluble oils.

## 2. Contact allergic eczema

This is a type IV allergic reaction which affects the few people who become sensitized to a particular allergen. The rash occurs at the site of contact with the allergen, but on the hands it is difficult to predict the cause from the site involved because the hands come into contact with so many things during the day. Nevertheless there are several well recognized patterns:

1  Finger tips — from *formalin* in laboratory workers and secretaries (from formaldehyde resins in cardboard folders), *local anaesthetics* in dentists, *garlic and onion* in cooks and less commonly *Balsam of Peru* in orange peel.

2  Centre of palm and flexor aspects of fingers — from *rubber*, *nickel* or *plastic* handle grips.

3  Whole hand, palm, dorsum and wrist — from *rubber* gloves.

4  Flexor aspect of wrist in lines — from the leaves of the indoor primula plant (*Primula obconica*) (see p. 43).

It is probably wise to patch test anyone with hand eczema who does not get better with topical steroids.

Contact allergic eczema may develop explosively with vesicles, exudate and crusting. If it develops more slowly then the rash is a poorly defined red scaly rash just like eczema elsewhere.

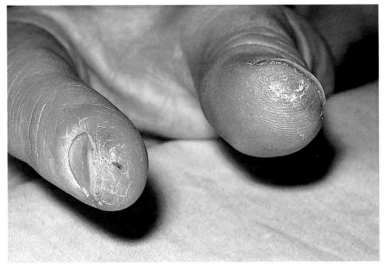

8.8 Contact allergic eczema in a dentist due to local anaesthetic paste.

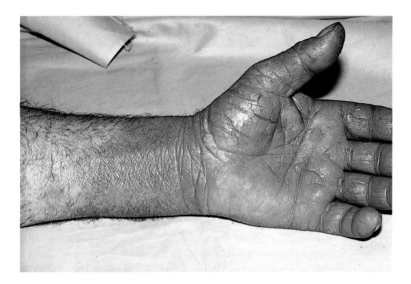

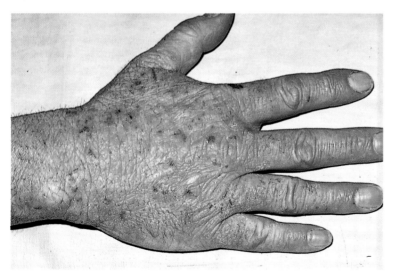

### Endogenous eczema

Endogenous eczema can occur on both the palms and dorsum of the hand. You should think of this diagnosis if the patient has symmetrical eczema, particularly if there is a past history of atopic eczema in childhood. The eczema is itchy and continual scratching will lead to *lichenification*. If it becomes secondarily infected with bacteria (staphylococci), pustules may occur. On the palms this differs from pustular psoriasis because all the pustules are the

*Left above*
**8.9** Contact allergic eczema due to rubber gloves: the eczema extends up the wrist to the level of the rubber glove.

*Left below*
**8.10** Lichenified eczema on the back of the hand.

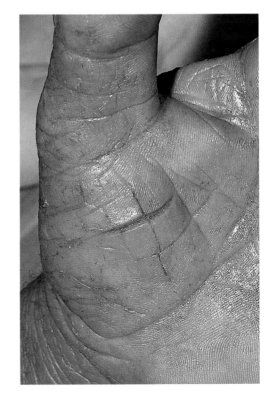

*Right*
**8.11** Endogenous eczema with fissures.

same colour. If *hyperkeratosis* occurs, it may split over the finger joints and along skin creases causing painful fissures.

## Discoid eczema

This is the only kind of eczema where the plaques are well circumscribed. There is usually obvious vesiculation and crusting on a red scaly base. In young adults the commonest site is the dorsum of the hands and fingers. In older individuals it is more usual on the lower legs.

**8.12** Discoid eczema.

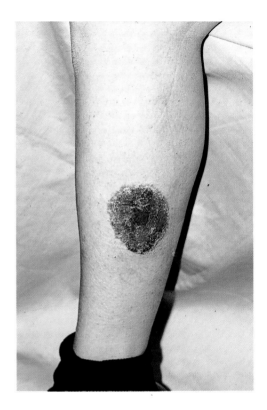

**Dorsum fingers/hand/forearm**
**Non-erythematous lesions**
**Surface normal**
**Skin coloured**

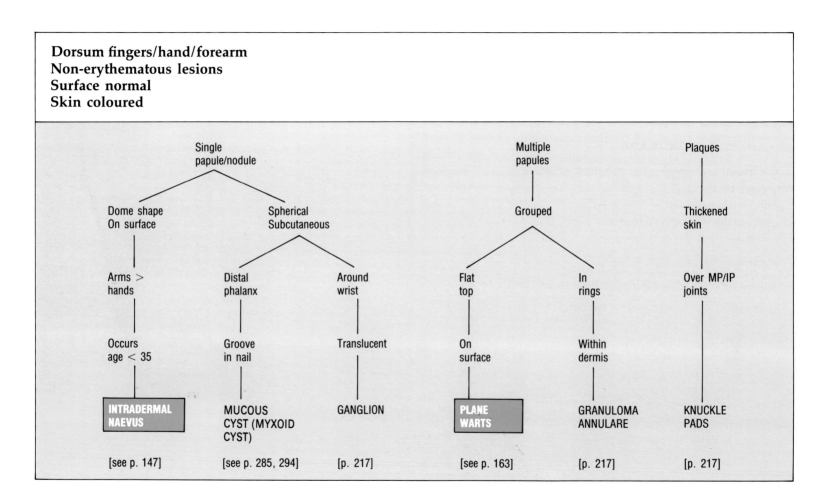

Single
papule/nodule

Dome shape
On surface

Spherical
Subcutaneous

Multiple
papules

Grouped

Plaques

Thickened
skin

Arms >
hands

Distal
phalanx

Around
wrist

Flat
top

In
rings

Over MP/IP
joints

Occurs
age < 35

Groove
in nail

Translucent

On
surface

Within
dermis

INTRADERMAL
NAEVUS

MUCOUS
CYST (MYXOID
CYST)

GANGLION

PLANE
WARTS

GRANULOMA
ANNULARE

KNUCKLE
PADS

[see p. 147]

[see p. 285, 294]

[p. 217]

[see p. 163]

[p. 217]

[p. 217]

## GANGLION (SYNOVIAL CYST)

This is a skin coloured nodule that occurs over the dorsum of the wrist or interphalangeal joints. It is attached to the tendon sheath or joint capsule.

## GRANULOMA ANNULARE

In this condition, small skin coloured or mauvish-pink papules form rings on the dorsum of the fingers, hand or foot. It is usually asymptomatic although it can be tender if knocked. It is harmless and eventually disappears spontaneously. The cause is unknown. It is distinguished from ringworm by not being scaly.

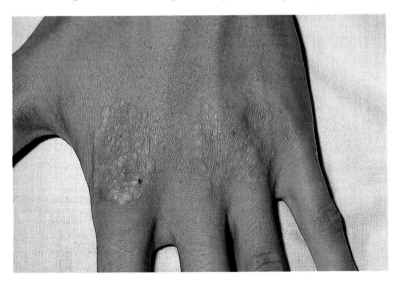

**8.13** Granuloma annulare.

## KNUCKLE PADS

This is a condition of young adults where thickened plaques appear over the knuckles or interphalangeal joints for no apparent reason.

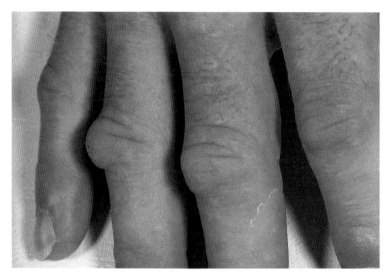

**8.14** Knuckle pads.

**Dorsum of hand and forearm**
**Non-erythematous lesions**
**Normal/warty/keratin surface**
**Brown colour**

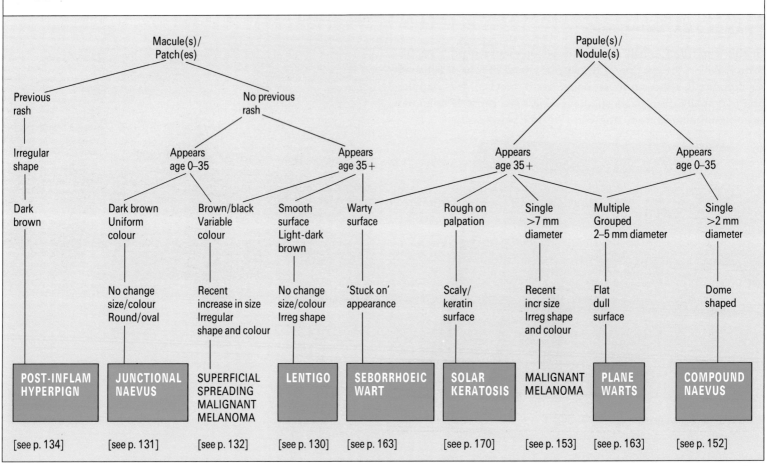

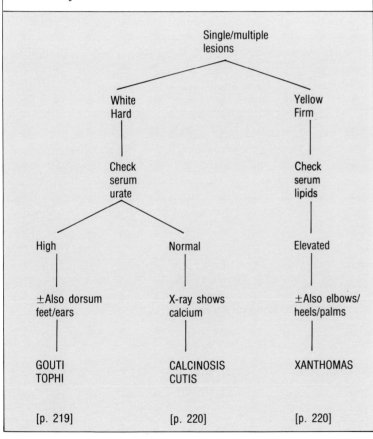

Fingers/hand/wrist
**Non-erythematous lesions**
**Surface normal**
**Colour yellow/white**

Single/multiple
lesions

White
Hard

Check
serum
urate

High

±Also dorsum
feet/ears

GOUTI
TOPHI

[p. 219]

Normal

X-ray shows
calcium

CALCINOSIS
CUTIS

[p. 220]

Yellow
Firm

Check
serum
lipids

Elevated

±Also elbows/
heels/palms

XANTHOMAS

[p. 220]

## GOUTY TOPHI

These are hard white or cream coloured papules or plaques due to deposition of sodium urate crystals in the dermis. Classically they occur on the helix or antihelix of the ear (see Fig. 9.28, p. 259), but occasionally are found on the dorsum of the hands and feet. Patients with tophi are likely to suffer from gout.

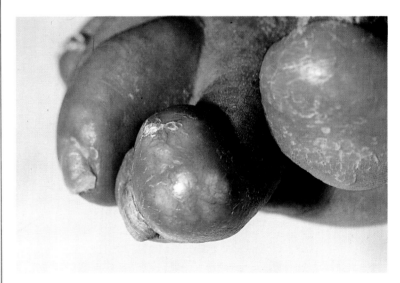

**8.15** Gouti tophi of the toes.

## CALCINOSIS CUTIS

These are hard white papules or plaques on the extremities which show up on X-rays. Classically they occur in scleroderma and dermatomyositis: they may be present in a patient who is otherwise well.

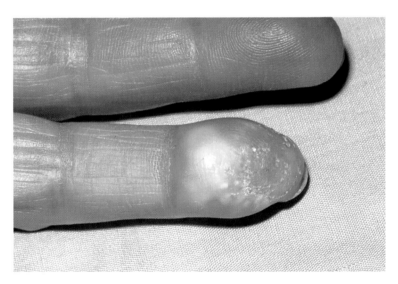

**8.16** Calcinosis cutis in a patient with scleroderma.

## XANTHOMA

These are lipid deposits in the skin, and may occur as yellow papules or nodules on the palms, elbows, knees or soles in association with a hyperlipidaemia.

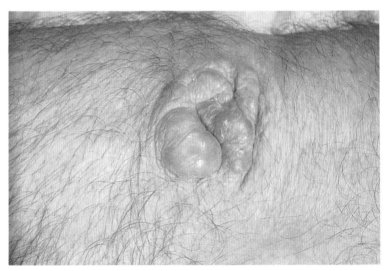

**8.17** Tuberose xanthoma on elbow.

**Dorsum of hand and forearm**
**Non-erythematous lesions**
**Horny/keratin/rough surface**
**Papules, plaques and nodules**

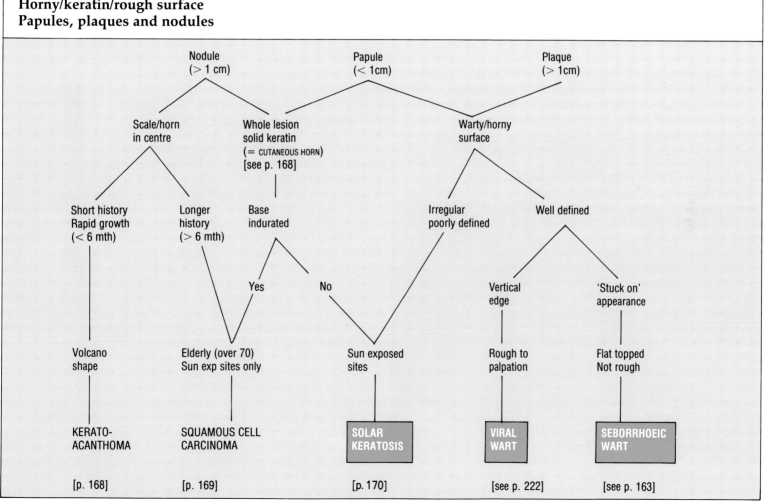

## VIRAL WARTS

Warts are an infection of the epidermis with one of the numerous human papilloma viruses. They are transmitted from one individual to another through broken skin (cuts, grazes etc.). They disappear spontaneously without scarring after weeks to years (average about 2 ¼ years) when the body has built up enough cell mediated immunity. Unfortunately immunity to one type of wart virus does not confer immunity to any of the others, i.e. having had an infection with the common wart virus does not prevent infection with the plantar wart or plane wart virus.

*Common warts* occur on the fingers, palm and dorsum of the hand. They are easily recognized as firm, rough, skin coloured or brown papules with black pin point dots on the surface.

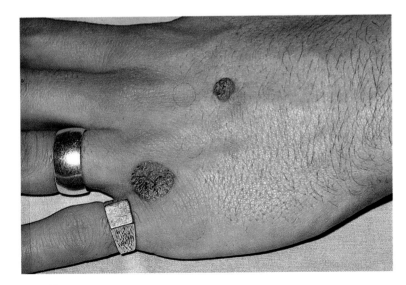

**8.18** Common warts.

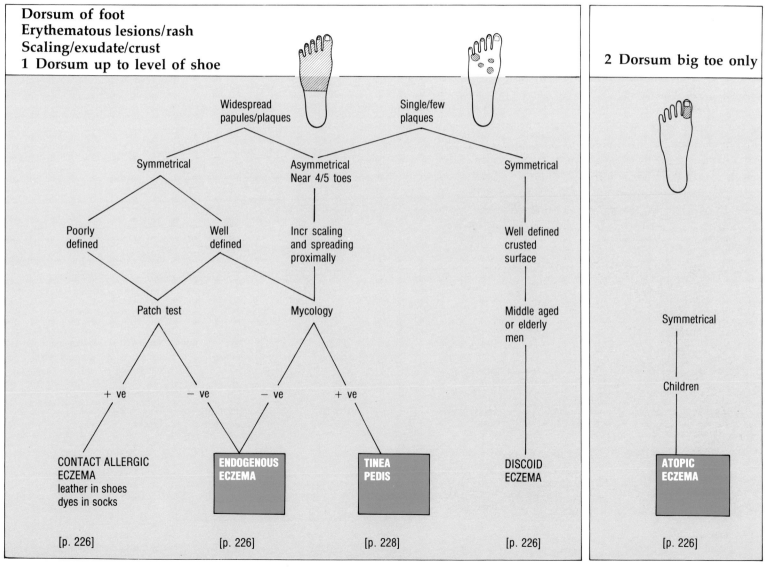

Dorsum of foot
Erythematous lesions/rash
Scaling/exudate/crust
1 Dorsum up to level of shoe

2 Dorsum big toe only

Widespread
papules/plaques

Single/few
plaques

Symmetrical

Asymmetrical
Near 4/5 toes

Symmetrical

Poorly
defined

Well
defined

Incr scaling
and spreading
proximally

Well defined
crusted
surface

Patch test

Mycology

Middle aged
or elderly
men

Symmetrical

Children

+ ve    − ve    − ve    + ve

CONTACT ALLERGIC
ECZEMA
leather in shoes
dyes in socks

ENDOGENOUS
ECZEMA

TINEA
PEDIS

DISCOID
ECZEMA

ATOPIC
ECZEMA

[p. 226]

[p. 226]

[p. 228]

[p. 226]

[p. 226]

**Erythematous/non-erythematous lesions**
**Soles**
**Widespread scaling/hyperkeratosis ± vesicles/pustules/maceration**
**1 Instep and weight bearing areas**

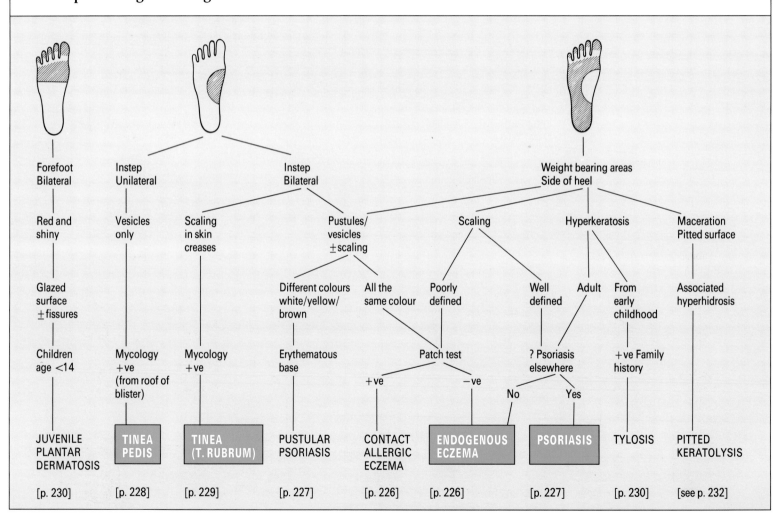

| | | | | | | | | |
|---|---|---|---|---|---|---|---|---|
| Forefoot Bilateral | Instep Unilateral | | Instep Bilateral | | Weight bearing areas Side of heel | | | |

Forefoot Bilateral

Red and shiny

Glazed surface ± fissures

Children age <14

JUVENILE PLANTAR DERMATOSIS

[p. 230]

Instep Unilateral

Vesicles only

Mycology +ve (from roof of blister)

**TINEA PEDIS**

[p. 228]

Scaling in skin creases

Mycology +ve

**TINEA (T. RUBRUM)**

[p. 229]

Instep Bilateral

Pustules/ vesicles ± scaling

Different colours white/yellow/ brown

Erythematous base

PUSTULAR PSORIASIS

[p. 227]

All the same colour

Patch test

+ve

CONTACT ALLERGIC ECZEMA

[p. 226]

Scaling

Poorly defined

−ve

No

**ENDOGENOUS ECZEMA**

[p. 226]

Weight bearing areas Side of heel

Hyperkeratosis

Well defined

? Psoriasis elsewhere

Yes

Adult

**PSORIASIS**

[p. 227]

From early childhood

+ve Family history

TYLOSIS

[p. 230]

Maceration Pitted surface

Associated hyperhidrosis

PITTED KERATOLYSIS

[see p. 232]

# Soles
## Scaling/vesicles/maceration
## 2  Between the toes

Between 3/4 & 4/5 only

Peeling/
fissures/
maceration

Unilateral — Bilateral

**Unilateral:**

All round
toe cleft

Circular
firm area

Mycology
+ ve

Hard keratin
underneath

**TINEA PEDIS** [p. 228]

**SOFT CORN** [p. 230]

**Bilateral:**

Wood's light

Pink
fluorescence — Negative

Gram stain
of skin scales

Gram +ve
diphtheroids

ERYTHRASMA [p. 228]

Direct
microscopy
of skin scales

Spores and
hyphae — Hyphae
only

**CANDIDA** [p. 228]

**TINEA PEDIS** [p. 228]

Between all toes

Scaly/
exudate/vesicles
erythematous

Bilateral

Well
defined

Poorly
defined

Psoriasis
elsewhere

Eczema
elsewhere

**PSORIASIS** [p. 227]

**ECZEMA** [p. 226]

## ECZEMA ON THE FEET

A symmetrical red scaly rash on the foot in which vesicles have been present at some stage is likely to be eczema. On the *dorsum* of the feet, a rash up to the level of the shoe and sparing the toe webs is usually due to a contact allergic eczema caused by leather in the shoe uppers, or azo dyes in nylon socks. The same pattern can occur in endogenous eczema. When the dorsum of the big toe alone is affected in a child aged 7–10 years, the diagnosis is nearly always atopic eczema. Discoid eczema, as elsewhere (dorsum of hands and lower legs), is a well-defined round or oval red scaly plaque with obvious vesiculation and crusting.

Symmetrical eczema on the *weight bearing area* of the soles is due to contact allergic eczema until proven otherwise. It is usually due to rubber in the soles of shoes or the azo dyes in nylon socks. The diagnosis can be confirmed by patch testing (see p. 11). An identical rash can occur with endogenous eczema or psoriasis. Because of the thick layer of keratin on the soles, rashes are much more difficult to distinguish from one another at this site. Vesicles

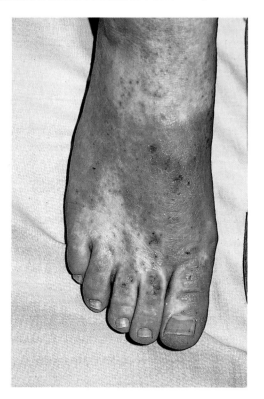

**8.19** Contact allergic eczema due to shoe leather.

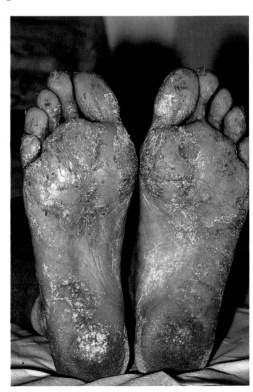

**8.20** Contact allergic eczema due to rubber in shoes. A similar pattern can occur in endogenous eczema and psoriasis.

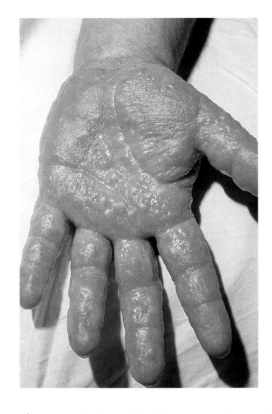

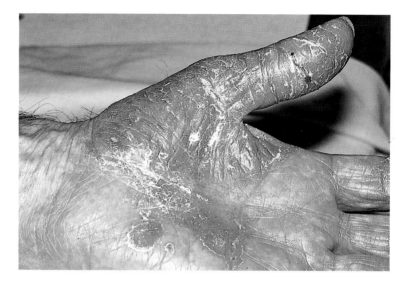

*Left*
**8.21** Pompholyx: vesicles on the palms and soles may stay intact for several days because of the thick stratum corneum.

often remain intact for days or weeks on the soles and look like tapioca. When they are present alone with no redness or scaling it is called *pompholyx*: this is usually a manifestation of endogenous or atopic eczema but can occur with tinea.

## PSORIASIS

Psoriasis of the hands and feet can be of three different patterns:
1  *Plaque psoriasis* is just like psoriasis elsewhere — well defined,

bright red, scaly plaques with silver scaling (Fig. 8.22).
2  *Hyperkeratosis* of the weight bearing area of the sole (Fig. 8.23). There is no redness to give you a clue to the diagnosis, but usually there is typical psoriasis elsewhere.
3  *Pustular psoriasis.* Here there are always pustules of different colours because each pustule dries out as it passes through the keratin layer changing in colour from white to yellow to orangey-brown to dark brown before peeling off in the scale (Fig. 8.24). There may or may not be a background redness and scaling. It differs from eczema or tinea which has become secondarily infected because in these conditions the pustules will all be of the same colour (there being no increased cell turnover of the epidermis in these conditions to push the pustules up through the keratin rapidly).

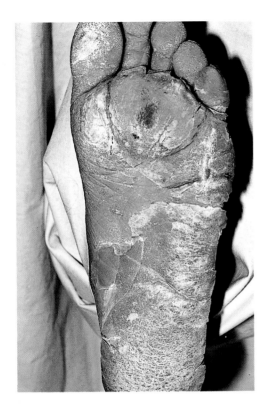

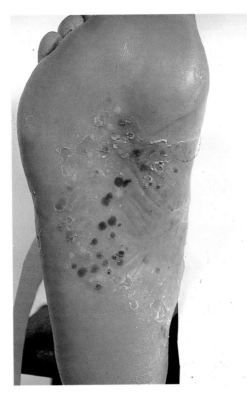

*Far left*
**8.23** Psoriasis on the sole: no erythema, just thick hyperkeratosis.

*Left*
**8.24** Pustular psoriasis of the sole: note the different coloured pustules. There is no erythema or scaling in this patient, although both can be present in this condition.

## TINEA PEDIS

There are four different patterns of tinea on the feet:

**1** The commonest is *scaling between the toes*, usually between the 4th and 5th toes where the toes are closest together and the humidity is highest. It begins on one foot only and the major symptom is itching. With time it may spread medially but rarely as far as the space between the 1st and 2nd toes. Later it may spread to the other foot and/or the toenails.

An identical scaly condition of the lateral toe spaces which is symmetrical from the start may be due to *erythrasma* or *candida*. To distinguish between these, first shine a Wood's light between the toes as erythrasma fluoresces bright pink. If there is no fluorescence, then take scrapings to examine under the microscope and for culture which will distinguish tinea from candida (see Figs. 1.1–1.4, pp. 9, 10)

**2** Less commonly a *scaly plaque will extend onto the dorsum of the foot* from the lateral toewebs.

**3** *Vesicles on the instep.* Unilateral vesicles are due to tinea until proven otherwise. Sometimes they may be present on both feet, but usually there will be much more on one foot than the other. The fungus will be found in the roof of the blisters, so cut off the roof with a pair of fine scissors to examine under the microscope or send for mycology culture.

**4** *White scaling on the soles.* This may be unilateral or bilateral, and is often associated with discolouration and thickening of the toenails: it is due to one particular fungus, *Trichophyton rubrum*. It may be found by chance when examining a patient's feet, or the patient may complain of burning or itching of the soles.

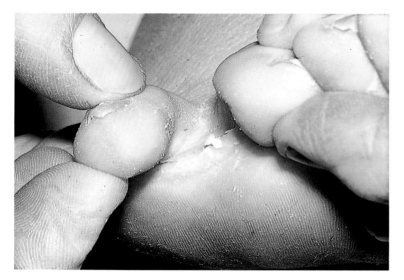

*Left*
**8.25** Scaling or maceration between the toes can be due to tinea, candida or erythrasma.

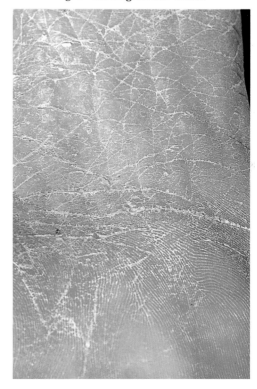

*Left*
**8.26** Vesicles on the instep due to tinea.

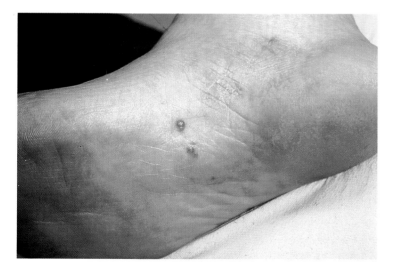

*Right*
**8.27** White scaling in the skin creases due to tinea (Trichophyton rubrum).

## TYLOSIS (PALMAR-PLANTAR KERATODERMA)

This is a genetically determined condition inherited as an autosomal dominant trait. Thickening of the keratin on the palms and soles is present from birth or early infancy. There are many variants of this condition, some with linear or punctate patterns.

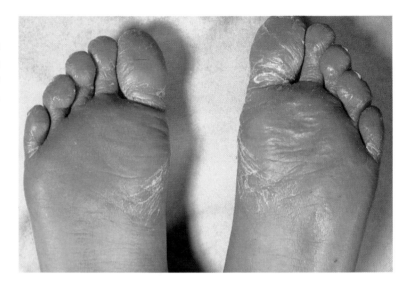

**8.29** Juvenile plantar dermatosis.

shiny, and children complain of itching or pain from fissures. It is thought to be due to modern footwear, nylon socks and synthetic soles which do not allow sweat to escape through the shoe. It gets better spontaneously after puberty.

## SOFT CORNS

Scaling between the 4th and 5th toes on one foot may be due to a soft corn. If you remove the surface keratin with a scalpel you will quickly come to firmer keratin underneath just like a corn elsewhere. Soft corns are due to wearing shoes that are too tight around the toes. The problem can be explained very simply to the patient by making them stand on a piece of paper on the floor in their bare feet. Draw around the affected foot with a pencil and then put their shoe on the drawing. It will be immediately obvious that the shoe is too small for the foot.

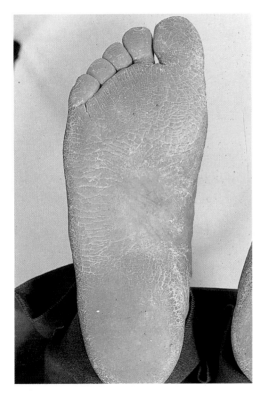

**8.28** Tylosis.

## JUVENILE PLANTAR DERMATOSIS

This condition occurs only in children, usually between the ages of 7 and 14. The plantar surface of the forefoot is bright red and

## Discrete non-erythematous lesions

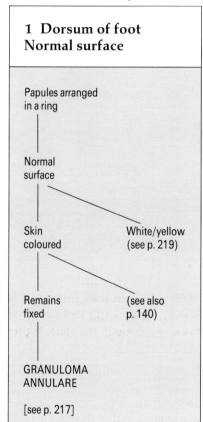

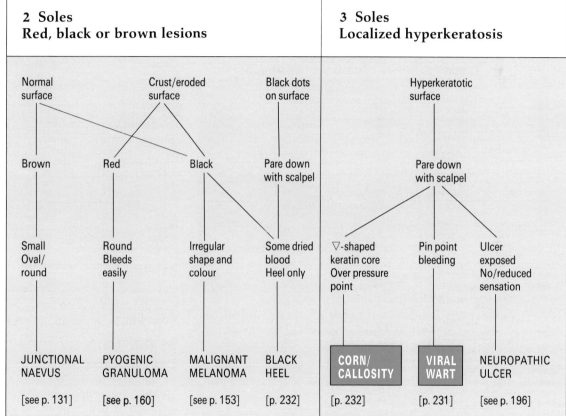

| 1 Dorsum of foot Normal surface | 2 Soles Red, black or brown lesions | 3 Soles Localized hyperkeratosis |
|---|---|---|

**1 Dorsum of foot — Normal surface**

Papules arranged in a ring → Normal surface → Skin coloured / White/yellow (see p. 219) → Remains fixed / (see also p. 140)

GRANULOMA ANNULARE

[see p. 217]

**2 Soles — Red, black or brown lesions**

Normal surface — Brown — Small Oval/round — JUNCTIONAL NAEVUS [see p. 131]

Crust/eroded surface — Red — Round Bleeds easily — PYOGENIC GRANULOMA [see p. 160]

Black — Irregular shape and colour — MALIGNANT MELANOMA [see p. 153]

Black dots on surface — Pare down with scalpel — Some dried blood Heel only — BLACK HEEL [p. 232]

**3 Soles — Localized hyperkeratosis**

Hyperkeratotic surface — Pare down with scalpel

▽-shaped keratin core Over pressure point — **CORN/ CALLOSITY** [p. 232]

Pin point bleeding — **VIRAL WART** [p. 231]

Ulcer exposed No/reduced sensation — NEUROPATHIC ULCER [see p. 196]

## VIRAL WART (VERRUCA)

Verruca is the proper name for a wart. Common warts on the hands are called verruca vulgaris and those on the feet verruca plantaris. In common usage, warts on the hands are called warts and those on the feet verrucas.

Individual lesions are discrete, round papules with a rough surface surrounded by a collar of hyperkeratosis. They may be very numerous and join together to form mosaic warts. If the diagnosis is in doubt, pare down the surface with a scalpel and very soon tiny bleeding points will be seen (Fig. 8.32).

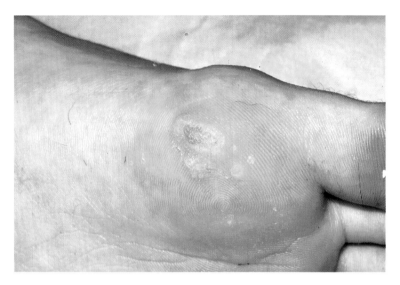

**8.30** Plantar warts.

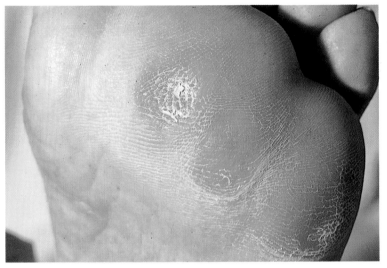

**8.31** Corns.

Two problems arise from warts on the feet.
1   They hurt. This is not due to the wart growing into the foot when it is situated on weight bearing areas, but to the hyperkeratosis that occurs around the wart. This grows outward and causes pain just as a stone in the shoe does. Paring the hyperkeratosis down with a pumice stone or scalpel will stop the pain. Less commonly the pain is excruciating due to thrombosis in the blood vessels in the wart. The wart goes black and within a few days drops off. Pain in this instance needs treating with analgesics.
2.   Children with verrucas are not allowed to swim. This may be overome by wearing a sock over the affected foot to prevent the spread of virus from one person to another.

## CORN

A corn is localized ▽-shaped area of hyperkeratosis over a pressure point on the foot. When pared down with scalpel no bleeding points are seen (Fig. 8.32).

## BLACK HEEL

It is quite common for bleeding to occur into the skin on the back of the heel in teenagers and young adults engaged in sporting activities, due to rubbing from shoes or direct trauma. A painless, dark red or black plaque is seen over the heel. when pared down with a scalpel, dried blood is seen within the keratin.

## PITTED KERATOLYSIS

The surface of the soles becomes eroded with shallow pits in the surface keratin. It occurs in individuals with hyperhidrosis of the feet and is due to colonization by a *Propionibacterium.*

**8.32** Differentiation between plantar wart and corn by paring down surface keratin.

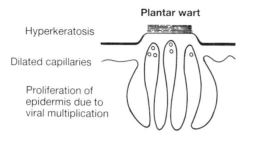

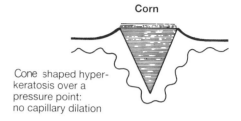

**Plantar wart**

Hyperkeratosis

Dilated capillaries

Proliferation of epidermis due to viral multiplication

Paring down produces pin-point bleeding

**Corn**

Cone shaped hyper-keratosis over a pressure point: no capillary dilation

Paring down produces a decreasing cone of keratin

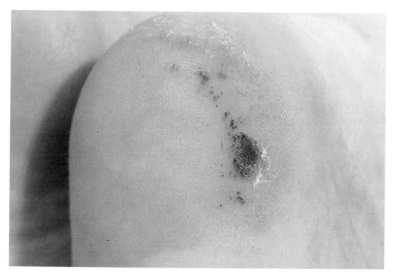

**8.33** Black heel.

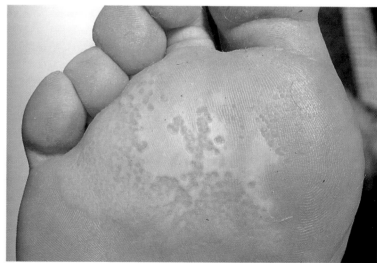

**8.34** Pitted keratolysis of the sole.

# Chapter 9
# Mouth, Tongue, Lips and Ear

## LESIONS AFFECTING THE MOUTH

**Mouth ulcers**
**1 Single ulcer or erosion**

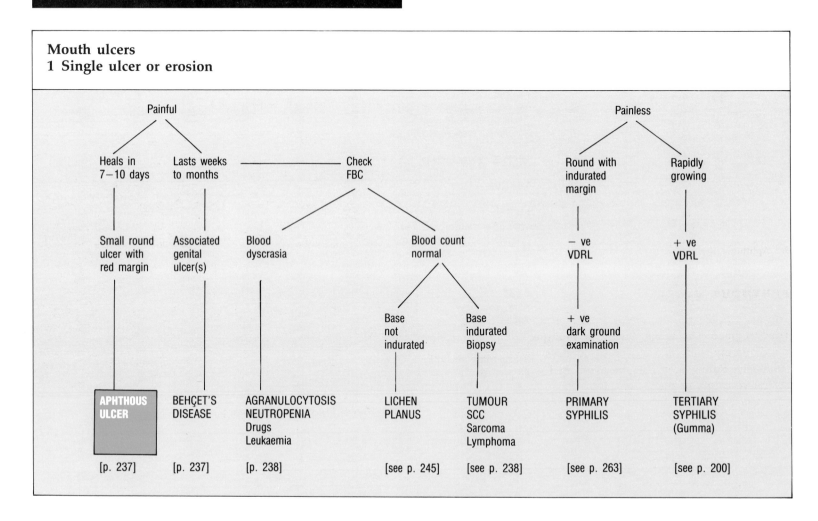

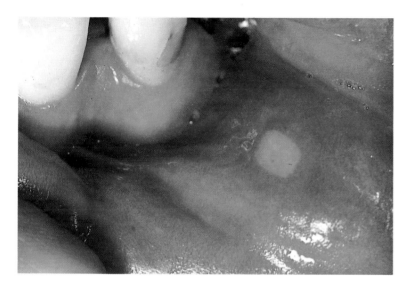

**9.1** Aphthous ulcer.

## APHTHOUS ULCERS

These are by far the commonest cause of recurrent mouth ulcers. They begin in the teens. Single or multiple round ulcers have a red margin and tend to last 7–10 days before healing spontaneously. Rarely they may be associated with Crohn's disease, ulcerative colitis or coeliac disease.

## BEHÇET'S DISEASE

A rare condition affecting mainly young men. You should think of it in any patient with recurrent oral and genital ulceration. The ulcers tend to be larger, deeper and longer lasting than aphthous ulcers. There will also be one or more of the following: iritis, arthritis, thrombophlebitis, sterile pustules on the skin, erythema nodosum and meningo-encephalitis. Such patients should be referred to hospital for treatment.

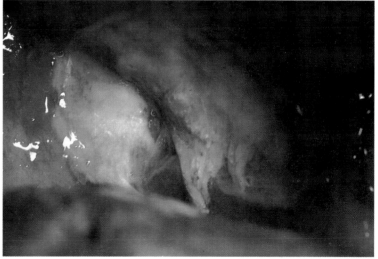

**9.2** Behçet's disease: ulcer on hard palate.

## BLOOD DYSCRASIAS

Agranulocytosis and neutropenia may result in mouth ulcers. These may be the first manifestation of leukaemia or be a side effect of drugs such as methotrexate.

## TUMOURS

A chronic ulcer where the blood count is normal may be due to an underlying tumour such as a squamous cell carcinoma (see Fig. 9.3), lymphoma, sarcoma or adenocarcinoma. A biopsy will be diagnostic.

**9.4** Primary herpes simplex infection of palate.

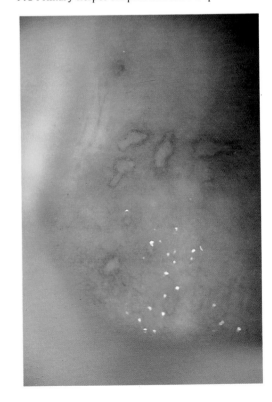

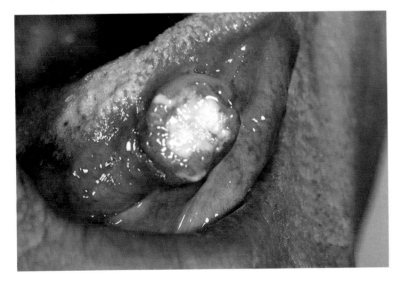

**9.3** Squamous cell carcinoma of tongue.

## Mouth ulcers
## 2 Multiple blisters/erosions/ulcers
### a Single acute episode

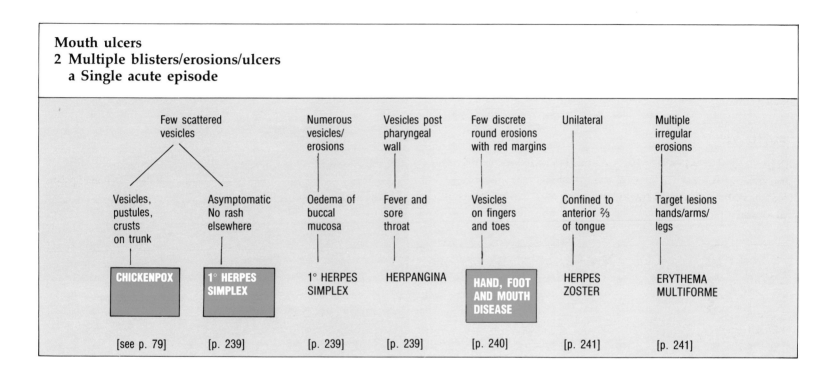

| Few scattered vesicles | | Numerous vesicles/ erosions | Vesicles post pharyngeal wall | Few discrete round erosions with red margins | Unilateral | Multiple irregular erosions |
|---|---|---|---|---|---|---|
| Vesicles, pustules, crusts on trunk | Asymptomatic No rash elsewhere | Oedema of buccal mucosa | Fever and sore throat | Vesicles on fingers and toes | Confined to anterior ⅔ of tongue | Target lesions hands/arms/ legs |
| CHICKENPOX | 1° HERPES SIMPLEX | 1° HERPES SIMPLEX | HERPANGINA | HAND, FOOT AND MOUTH DISEASE | HERPES ZOSTER | ERYTHEMA MULTIFORME |
| [see p. 79] | [p. 239] | [p. 239] | [p. 239] | [p. 240] | [p. 241] | [p. 241] |

## PRIMARY HERPES SIMPLEX

Most primary infections with the herpes simplex virus occur in early childhood and are asymptomatic. Occasionally they may cause an acute gingivostomatitis with fever and general malaise.

## HERPANGINA

This is an infection with a Coxsackie virus. It differs from herpes simplex in involving the posterior pharyngeal wall and is associated with fever and sore throat.

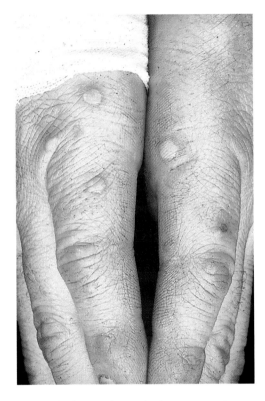

**9.5** Hand, foot and mouth disease: vesicles on fingers.

*Right above*
**9.6** Hand, foot and mouth disease.

*Right below*
**9.7** Erythema multi-forme: mouth erosions.

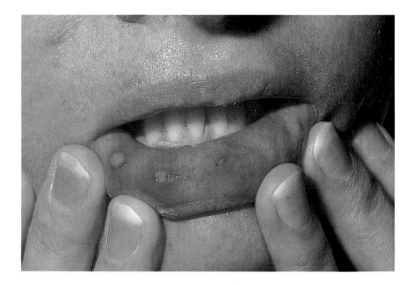

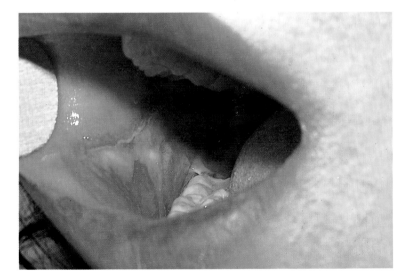

## HAND, FOOT AND MOUTH DISEASE

This is a mild Coxsackie infection where a few round erosions with a red margin are seen in the mouth. They look like small aphthous ulcers but are associated with small grey blisters with a red halo on the fingers and toes.

## HERPES ZOSTER

Herpes zoster involving the mandibular branch of the Vth cranial nerve is uncommon, but presents with unilateral vesicles on the anterior two-thirds of the tongue as well as the characteristic vesicles on the chin.

## STEVENS–JOHNSON SYNDROME

Erythema multiforme involving the mucous membranes presents with multiple irregular erosions. Extensive involvement of the mouth, lips, conjunctivae and genitalia is called the Stevens–Johnson syndrome, and carries a significant mortality. The causes of this are the same as for ordinary erythema multiforme (see p. 208).

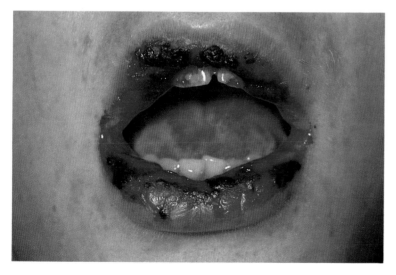

**9.8** Stevens-Johnson syndrome.

---

**Mouth ulcers**
**2 Multiple blisters/erosions/ulcers**
  **b Recurrent acute episodes**

Small round ulcers with red margins

Large blisters/ erosions

Irregular erosions

Always same site ± similar lesions body

Not always same site

Associated target lesions

**APHTHOUS ULCERS**

**FIXED DRUG ERUPTION**

**DRUG SIDE EFFECTS** Cytotoxics

**ERYTHEMA MULTIFORME** due to herpes simplex

[see p. 237]    [see p. 134]    [see p. 238]    [see p. 241]

## Mouth ulcers
## 2 Multiple blisters/erosions/ulcers
### c Chronic erosions/ulcers

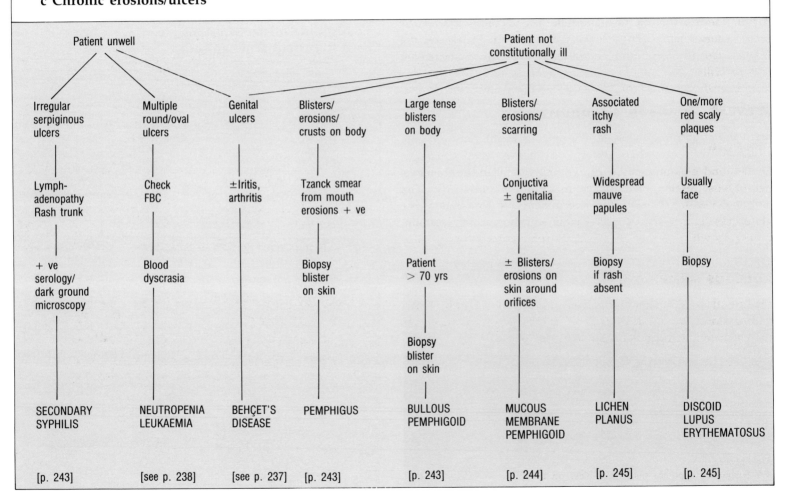

Patient unwell

Patient not constitutionally ill

| Irregular serpiginous ulcers | Multiple round/oval ulcers | Genital ulcers | Blisters/ erosions/ crusts on body | Large tense blisters on body | Blisters/ erosions/ scarring | Associated itchy rash | One/more red scaly plaques |
|---|---|---|---|---|---|---|---|
| Lymph-adenopathy Rash trunk | Check FBC | ±Iritis, arthritis | Tzanck smear from mouth erosions + ve | | Conjuctiva ± genitalia | Widespread mauve papules | Usually face |
| + ve serology/ dark ground microscopy | Blood dyscrasia | | Biopsy blister on skin | Patient > 70 yrs | ± Blisters/ erosions on skin around orifices | Biopsy if rash absent | Biopsy |
| | | | | Biopsy blister on skin | | | |
| SECONDARY SYPHILIS | NEUTROPENIA LEUKAEMIA | BEHÇET'S DISEASE | PEMPHIGUS | BULLOUS PEMPHIGOID | MUCOUS MEMBRANE PEMPHIGOID | LICHEN PLANUS | DISCOID LUPUS ERYTHEMATOSUS |
| [p. 243] | [see p. 238] | [see p. 237] | [p. 243] | [p. 243] | [p. 244] | [p. 245] | [p. 245] |

## SECONDARY SYPHILIS

Irregular serpiginous ulcers occur on the buccal mucosa and tongue in secondary syphilis. These lesions are highly infectious and the treponemes may be found on dark ground microscopy. Other features will be present such as general malaise, lymphadenopathy, a rash on the trunk (p. 112), palms and soles, and warty lesions around the anus.

## PEMPHIGUS

Blisters and erosions in the mouth are usually the first sign of pemphigus. The diagnosis can be made by scraping the base of an erosion with a blunt scalpel and putting the scrapings onto a glass slide (Tzanck smear); a PAP stain will show round (acantholytic) cells which are diagnostic of pemphigus (see also p. 122).

## BULLOUS PEMPHIGOID

The mouth is occasionally involved in pemphigoid with blisters and erosions on the buccal mucosa. The diagnosis is made from the characteristic blisters on the skin (see p. 123).

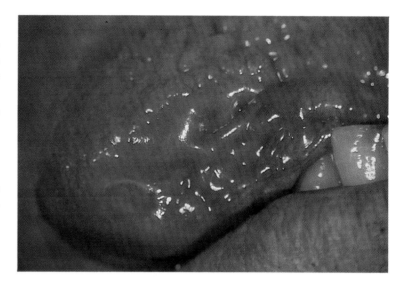

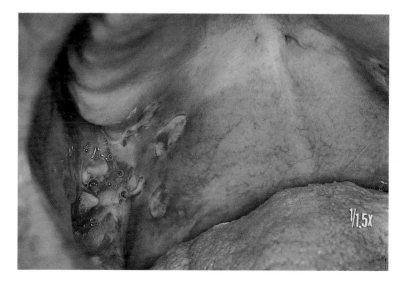

*Right above*
**9.9** Secondary syphilis: snail track ulcer on the tongue.

*Right below*
**9.10** Ulceration in the mouth due to pemphigus.

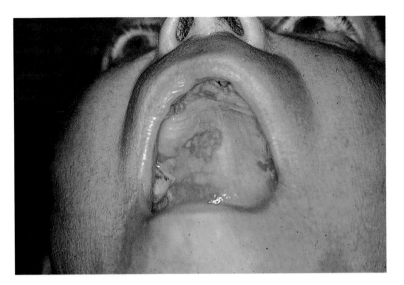

## MUCOUS MEMBRANE PEMPHIGOID

This is a rare autoimmune disease in which antibody against the basement membrane of the epidermis is found. Mucous membranes (mouth, eyes and genitalia) are predominantly involved with blisters, erosions and scarring. Blisters can also occur on the skin adjacent to orifices. The diagnosis is usually made by looking at the eyes; scarring and adhesions between the palpebral conjunctivae are characteristic.

*Left above*
**9.11** Mucous membrane pemphigoid: mouth erosions.

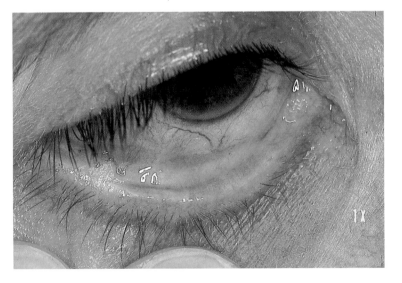

*Left below*
**9.12** Mocuous membrane pemphigoid: conjunctival adhesions.

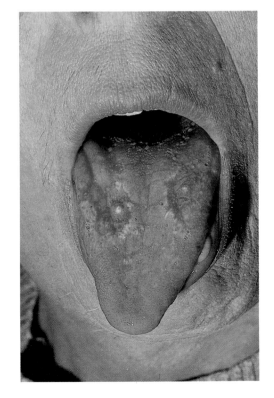

*Right*
**9.13** Lichen planus: painful ulceration.

## LICHEN PLANUS

Rarely, chronic ulceration of the mouth occurs in lichen planus. The edge of the ulcer is usually white. At the start there may have been the characteristic rash of lichen planus on the body (see p. 94), but ulceration in the mouth can go on for years and continue long after the rash is gone.

## DISCOID LUPUS ERYTHEMATOSUS

Discrete red erosions in the mouth may be present in discoid LE. The diagnosis is made from the typical skin lesions on the face (see p. 68).

**9.14** Candida.

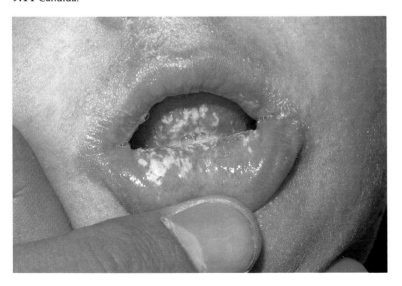

### Mouth lesions
### White/yellow

White papules/ plaques in mouth

Multiple (1mm) white/yellow macules/ papules

Remove with spatula — Adherent

Red base

Lacey pattern — Thick plaque — Along teeth line — Inside cheeks On lips

Mycology + ve

Mauve papules on trunk/limbs

Biopsy

**CANDIDA (Thrush)**

LICHEN PLANUS

LEUCOPLAKIA

**CHEEK BITING**

**FORDYCE SPOTS**

[p. 245]  [p. 246]  [p. 246]  [p. 246]  [p. 246]

## CANDIDA

Thrush occurs in the very young, the very old or those on antibiotics or cytotoxic drugs. White papules scrape off easily with a spatula to leave a red surface. If these are mixed with potassium hydroxide, the spores and hyphae are easily seen on direct microscopy (see Fig. 1.3, p. 10) or the organism can be cultured in 48 hours.

## LICHEN PLANUS

Lichen planus in the mouth is usually asymptomatic. If the typical mauve papular rash is seen elsewhere (p. 94), look in the mouth and in many cases the white criss-cross pattern will be seen on the buccal mucosa.

## CHEEK BITING

A fold of buccal mucous membrane is seen heaped up along the teeth line. It is quite harmless.

## FORDYCE SPOTS

These are small discrete white or yellow papules on the lips or buccal mucosa due to sebaceous gland hyperplasia. They are very common and completely harmless.

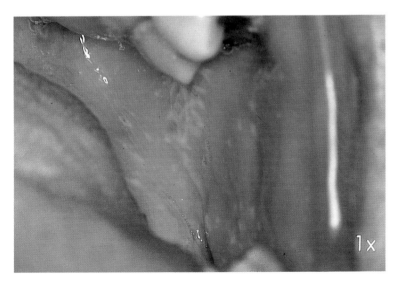

9.15 Lichen planus: asymptomatic lesions.

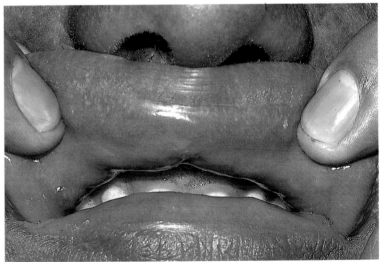

9.16 Fordyce spots due to sebaceous gland hyperplasia.

## LEUKOPLAKIA

This is a persistent white hyperkeratotic plaque in the mouth due to epithelial dysplasia or carcinoma-in-situ.

## ABNORMALITIES OF THE TONGUE

### SMOOTH TONGUE

A smooth tongue may be associated with iron deficiency, malabsorption or pernicious anaemia.

### FURRED TONGUE

This is a common condition due to hypertrophy of the filiform papillae, and is completely harmless.

### BLACK HAIRY TONGUE

This is due to hyperplasia of the filiform papillae which begins posteriorly and centrally. It is usually asymptomatic.

### FISSURED TONGUE (SCROTAL TONGUE)

Deep grooves in the tongue may be a congenital abnormality, or if seen together with facial nerve palsy and swelling of the lips indicates the Melkersson—Rosenthal syndrome.

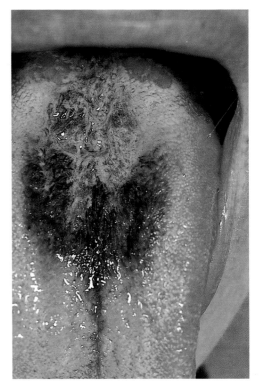

**9.17** Black hairy tongue.

## GEOGRAPHIC TONGUE

A very common benign condition where smooth red patches appear on the dorsum of the tongue giving a map-like appearance. These move about from day to day.

## LARGE TONGUE (MACROGLOSSIA)

The tongue may be large from birth or from early childhood in individuals with Down's syndrome, or with lymphangiomas, haemangiomas or neurofibromas of the tongue.

Intermittent enlargement of the tongue (lasting < 24 hours) is usually due to angio-oedema (see p. 36) and associated with urticaria. After middle age, enlargement of the tongue should make you think of amyloidosis.

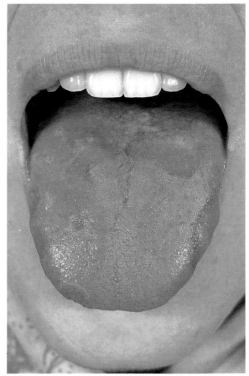

**9.18** Geographic tongue.

# ABNORMALITIES OF THE LIPS

## Lips
## 1 Vesicles/erosions/ulcers

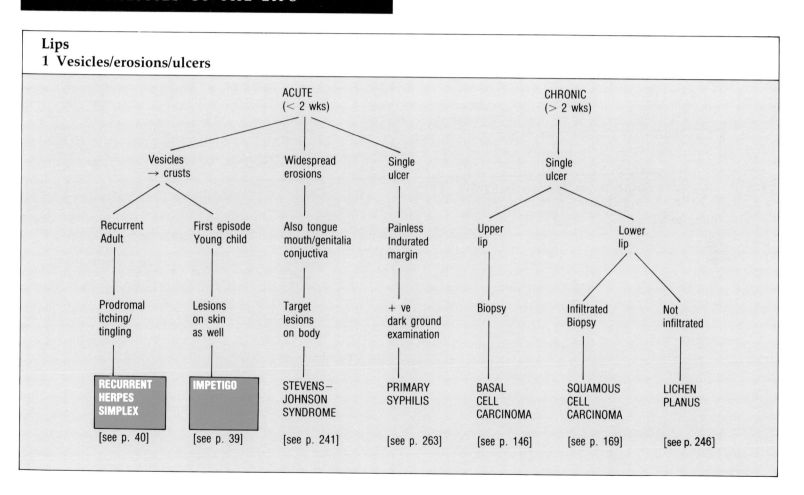

ACUTE (< 2 wks)

- Vesicles → crusts
  - Recurrent Adult
    - Prodromal itching/ tingling
      - **RECURRENT HERPES SIMPLEX**
      - [see p. 40]
  - First episode Young child
    - Lesions on skin as well
      - **IMPETIGO**
      - [see p. 39]
- Widespread erosions
  - Also tongue mouth/genitalia conjuctiva
    - Target lesions on body
      - STEVENS—JOHNSON SYNDROME
      - [see p. 241]
- Single ulcer
  - Painless Indurated margin
    - + ve dark ground examination
      - PRIMARY SYPHILIS
      - [see p. 263]

CHRONIC (> 2 wks)

- Single ulcer
  - Upper lip
    - Biopsy
      - BASAL CELL CARCINOMA
      - [see p. 146]
  - Lower lip
    - Infiltrated Biopsy
      - SQUAMOUS CELL CARCINOMA
      - [see p. 169]
    - Not infiltrated
      - LICHEN PLANUS
      - [see p. 246]

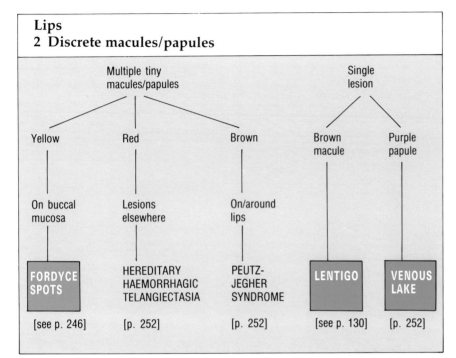

**Lips**
**2 Discrete macules/papules**

Multiple tiny macules/papules

Single lesion

Yellow

On buccal mucosa

**FORDYCE SPOTS**

[see p. 246]

Red

Lesions elsewhere

HEREDITARY HAEMORRHAGIC TELANGIECTASIA

[p. 252]

Brown

On/around lips

PEUTZ-JEGHER SYNDROME

[p. 252]

Brown macule

**LENTIGO**

[see p. 130]

Purple papule

**VENOUS LAKE**

[p. 252]

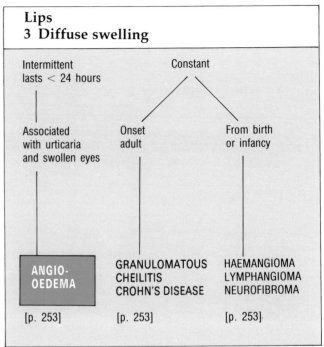

**Lips**
**3 Diffuse swelling**

Intermittent lasts < 24 hours

Constant

Associated with urticaria and swollen eyes

**ANGIO-OEDEMA**

[p. 253]

Onset adult

GRANULOMATOUS CHEILITIS CROHN'S DISEASE

[p. 253]

From birth or infancy

HAEMANGIOMA LYMPHANGIOMA NEUROFIBROMA

[p. 253]

## Lips
## 4 Erythematous/scaly/rough, papules/plaques/nodules

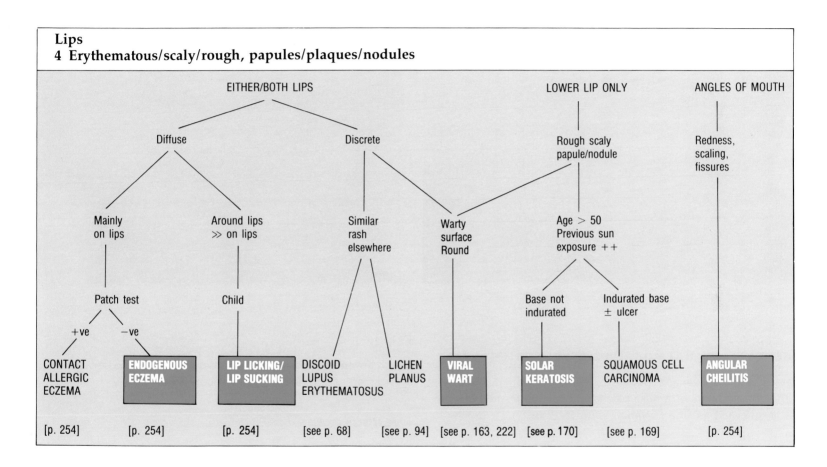

EITHER/BOTH LIPS

LOWER LIP ONLY

ANGLES OF MOUTH

Diffuse

Discrete

Rough scaly
papule/nodule

Redness,
scaling,
fissures

Mainly
on lips

Around lips
≫ on lips

Similar
rash
elsewhere

Warty
surface
Round

Age > 50
Previous sun
exposure + +

Patch test

Child

Base not
indurated

Indurated base
± ulcer

+ve    −ve

CONTACT
ALLERGIC
ECZEMA

**ENDOGENOUS
ECZEMA**

**LIP LICKING/
LIP SUCKING**

DISCOID
LUPUS
ERYTHEMATOSUS

LICHEN
PLANUS

**VIRAL
WART**

**SOLAR
KERATOSIS**

SQUAMOUS CELL
CARCINOMA

**ANGULAR
CHEILITIS**

[p. 254]    [p. 254]    [p. 254]    [see p. 68]    [see p. 94]    [see p. 163, 222]    [see p. 170]    [see p. 169]    [p. 254]

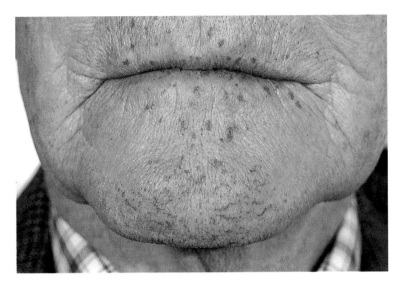

**9.19** Hereditary heamorrhagic telangiectasia.

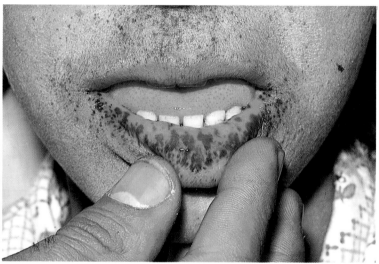

**9.20** Peutz-Jegher syndrome.

## HEREDITARY HAEMORRHAGIC TELANGIECTASIA

Small red macules and papules occur on the lips, tongue and fingers associated with nose bleeds and gastrointestinal bleeding. It is inherited as an autosomal dominant trait.

## PEUTZ-JEGHER SYNDROME

A rare genetically determined condition transmitted as an autosomal dominant trait. Brown macules and papules on the lips, skin around the mouth, fingers and toes occur in early childhood. These are associated with small bowel polyps.

## VENOUS LAKE

A solitary purple soft papule on the upper or lower lip is common in the middle aged or elderly.

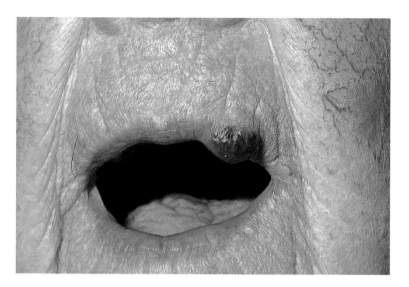

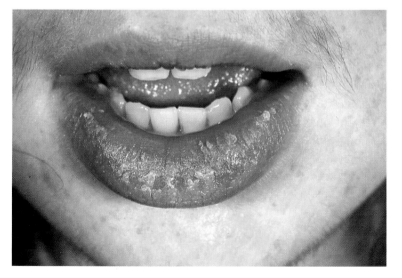

## ANGIO-OEDEMA

Urticaria affecting the lips, tongue and eyelids causes swelling more than redness; it is called angio-oedema. It will last less than 24 hours before starting to go down. It is usually associated with urticaria elsewhere (see p. 72).

## GRANULOMATOUS CHEILITIS

In granulomatous cheilitis the whole lip (upper or lower) is swollen. Initially this may fluctuate quite a lot, but eventually the swelling becomes permanent. The cause is unknown. If the buccal mucosa is also thickened, consider Crohn's disease which may be confirmed by biopsy. If there is an associated facial nerve palsy and/or scrotal tongue consider the Melkersson–Rosenthal syndrome.

## HAEMANGIOMA/LYMPHANGIOMA/NEUROFIBROMA

Any of these can occur on the lips and produce swelling which presents at birth or in early childhood and remains permanently.

*Left above*
**9.21** Venous lake.

*Left below*
**9.22** Granulomatous cheilitis.

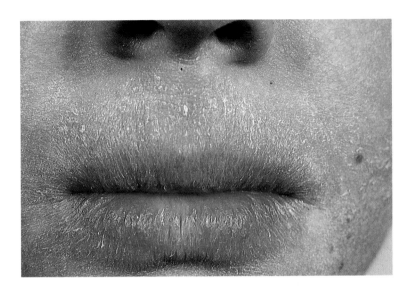

## ECZEMA ON THE LIPS

Contact allergic eczema can occur on the lips from lipstick, lip salves, toothpaste, or mouth washes. The diagnosis is confirmed by patch testing. Atopic eczema may affect the lips as well as the rest of the skin of the face (see p. 103). Many children suck or lick their lips causing a red scaly rash around the mouth which only extends as far as the tongue can reach.

## ANGULAR CHEILITIS

Cheilitis means inflammation of the lips, and in angular cheilitis only the corners of the lips are involved. It occurs in individuals who wear dentures, and is usually due to candida infection from under the top denture.

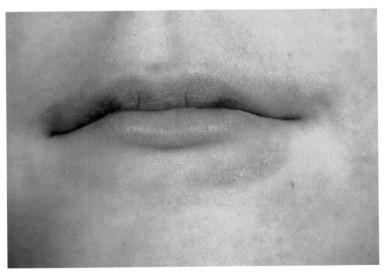

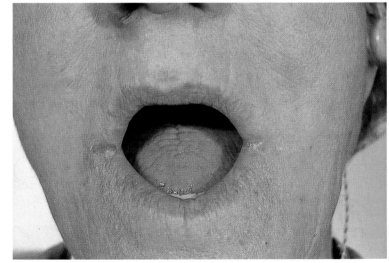

## LESIONS AFFECTING THE EARS

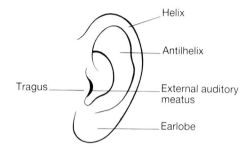

Helix

Antilhelix

External auditory meatus

Tragus

Earlobe

### 1 Helix and antihelix

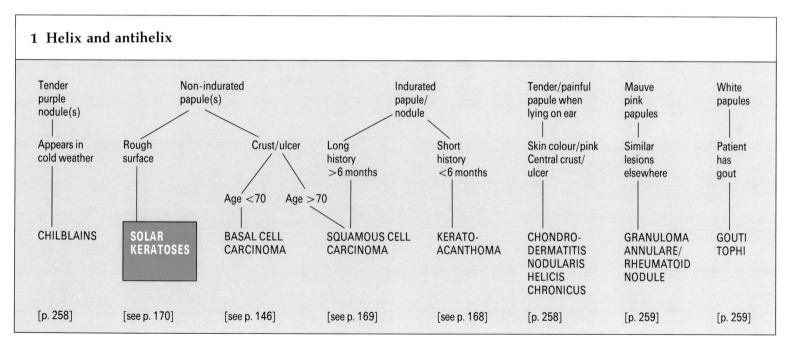

| Tender purple nodule(s) | | Non-indurated papule(s) | | | Indurated papule/ nodule | | Tender/painful papule when lying on ear | Mauve pink papules | White papules |
|---|---|---|---|---|---|---|---|---|---|
| Appears in cold weather | Rough surface | | Crust/ulcer | | Long history >6 months | Short history <6 months | Skin colour/pink Central crust/ ulcer | Similar lesions elsewhere | Patient has gout |
| | | | Age <70 | Age >70 | | | | | |
| CHILBLAINS | SOLAR KERATOSES | | BASAL CELL CARCINOMA | SQUAMOUS CELL CARCINOMA | | KERATO-ACANTHOMA | CHONDRO-DERMATITIS NODULARIS HELICIS CHRONICUS | GRANULOMA ANNULARE/ RHEUMATOID NODULE | GOUTI TOPHI |
| [p. 258] | [see p. 170] | | [see p. 146] | [see p. 169] | | [see p. 168] | [p. 258] | [p. 259] | [p. 259] |

*Facing page*
*Left above*
**9.23** Atopic eczema involving lips and skin around lips.

*Left below*
**9.24** Changes due to lip licking in an 8 year old boy.

*Right*
**9.25** Angular cheilitis.

**2 Around external meatus/in canal**

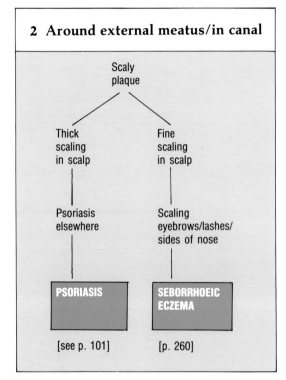

Scaly
plaque

Thick
scaling
in scalp

Fine
scaling
in scalp

Psoriasis
elsewhere

Scaling
eyebrows/lashes/
sides of nose

**PSORIASIS**

**SEBORRHOEIC
ECZEMA**

[see p. 101]

[p. 260]

**3 Earlobe**

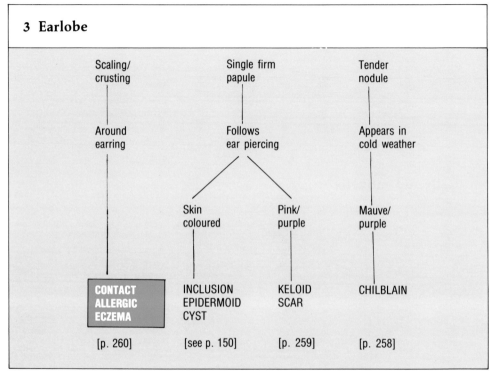

Scaling/
crusting

Single firm
papule

Tender
nodule

Around
earring

Follows
ear piercing

Appears in
cold weather

Skin
coloured

Pink/
purple

Mauve/
purple

**CONTACT
ALLERGIC
ECZEMA**

INCLUSION
EPIDERMOID
CYST

KELOID
SCAR

CHILBLAIN

[p. 260]

[see p. 150]

[p. 259]

[p. 258]

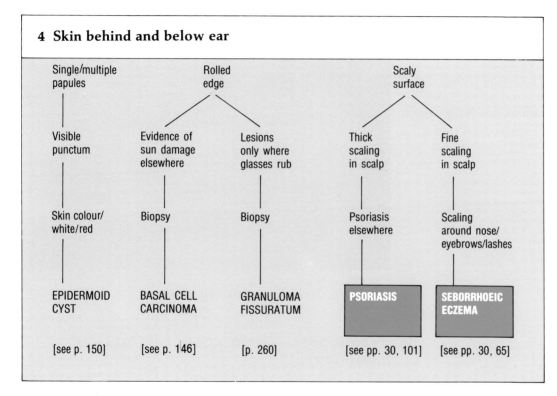

## 4 Skin behind and below ear

Single/multiple papules
↓
Visible punctum
↓
Skin colour/ white/red
↓
EPIDERMOID CYST
[see p. 150]

Rolled edge
↓
Evidence of sun damage elsewhere
↓
Biopsy
↓
BASAL CELL CARCINOMA
[see p. 146]

Lesions only where glasses rub
↓
Biopsy
↓
GRANULOMA FISSURATUM
[p. 260]

Scaly surface
↓
Thick scaling in scalp
↓
Psoriasis elsewhere
↓
PSORIASIS
[see pp. 30, 101]

Fine scaling in scalp
↓
Scaling around nose/ eyebrows/lashes
↓
SEBORRHOEIC ECZEMA
[see pp. 30, 65]

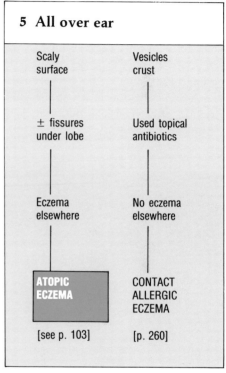

## 5 All over ear

Scaly surface
↓
± fissures under lobe
↓
Eczema elsewhere
↓
ATOPIC ECZEMA
[see p. 103]

Vesicles crust
↓
Used topical antibiotics
↓
No eczema elsewhere
↓
CONTACT ALLERGIC ECZEMA
[p. 260]

## CHILBLAINS

Tender, itchy, mauve papules and nodules on the earlobes and helix occur in cold weather and last up to 2 weeks. Similar lesions can occur on other exposed sites, e.g. fingers, toes, and nose. They occur in individuals who get very cold and warm up too quickly. The lesions are due to an abnormal reaction to cold when constriction of arterioles is followed by exudation of fluid into the tissues on rewarming.

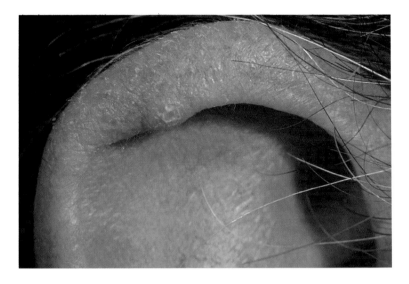

**9.27** Chondrodermatitis nodularis helicis chronicus.

## CHONDRODERMATITIS NODULARIS HELICIS CHRONICUS

This is a painful skin-coloured or pink papule on the helix or anti-helix; there may be a central area of scaling or crusting. The history of pain in bed at night when the patient lies on that side differentiates it from solar keratoses and skin tumours, which if painful, hurt all the time. It is a benign condition but the pain can be relieved by excising the lesion.

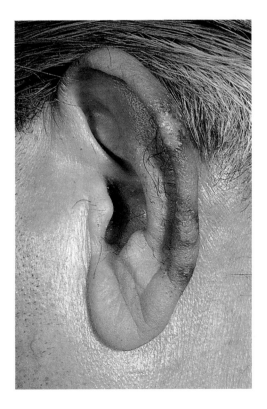

**9.26** Chilblains.

## GRANULOMA ANNULARE/RHEUMATOID NODULE

Pink or red papules on the antihelix will be one of these. A biopsy is necessary to make the diagnosis.

## GOUTI TOPHI

White papules on the antihelix are usually tophi (see p. 219).

## KELOID SCAR

A round pink/purple papule or nodule may develop on the ear lobe following ear piercing. It may gradually increase in size and become unsightly. It is differentiated from an inclusion epidermoid cyst (due to epidermis being implanted into the dermis at the time of ear piercing) by its colour.

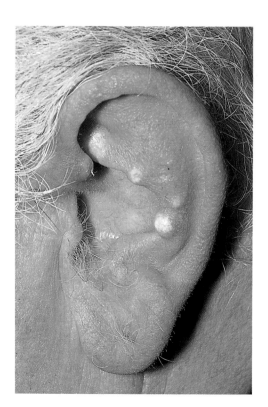

**9.28** Gouti tophi.

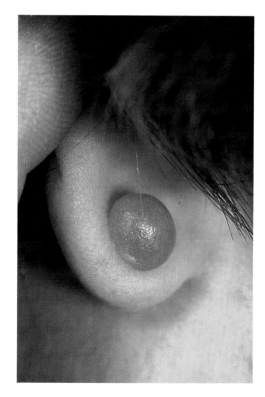

**9.29** Keloid scar from ear piercing.

## ECZEMA ON THE EAR

Eczema on the ear usually occurs in association with eczema elsewhere.

*Otitis externa*, i.e. eczema of the external auditary canal and meatus is usually due to seborrhoeic eczema, and there will be other evidence of this, e.g. scaling in the scalp (see pp. 30, 65).

*Contact allergic eczema* may occur on the earlobe from nickel in earrings; gold and silver do not usually cause allergy. Medicaments, especially antibiotics and antihistamines, affect the whole earlobe and external auditory canal causing an acute eczema with vesicles, exudate and crusting (see Fig. 2.25, p. 31).

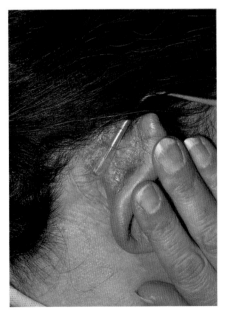

**9.30** Contact allergic eczema due to plastic of spectacles.

## GRANULOMA FISSURATUM

This occurs from the pressure of spectacles and occurs at the side of the bridge of the nose or behind the ear. It looks like a basal cell carcinoma, and is distinguished by skin biopsy.

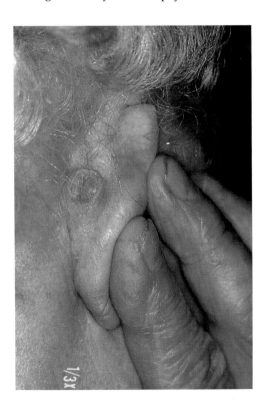

**9.31** Granuloma fissuratum.

# Chapter 10
# Genitalia

**Genital ulcers**
**1  Single ulcer**

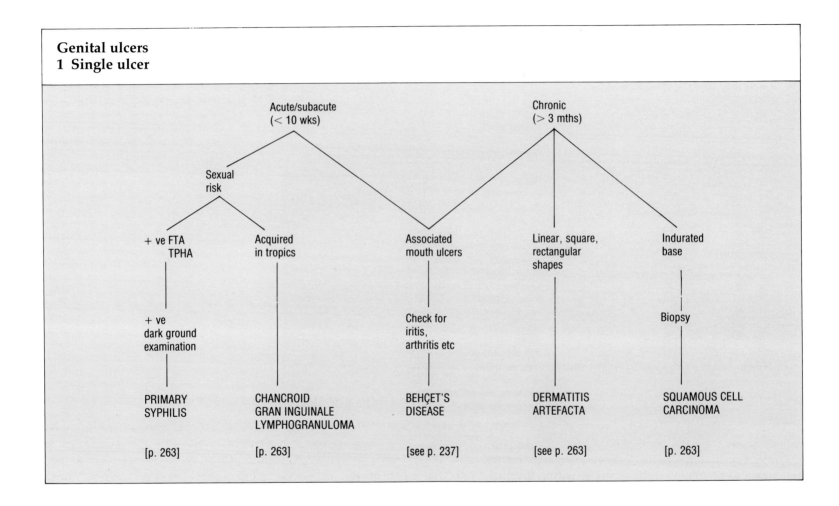

Acute/subacute
(< 10 wks)

Chronic
(> 3 mths)

Sexual
risk

+ ve FTA
TPHA

Acquired
in tropics

Associated
mouth ulcers

Linear, square,
rectangular
shapes

Indurated
base

+ ve
dark ground
examination

Check for
iritis,
arthritis etc

Biopsy

PRIMARY
SYPHILIS

CHANCROID
GRAN INGUINALE
LYMPHOGRANULOMA

BEHÇET'S
DISEASE

DERMATITIS
ARTEFACTA

SQUAMOUS CELL
CARCINOMA

[p. 263]

[p. 263]

[see p. 237]

[see p. 263]

[p. 263]

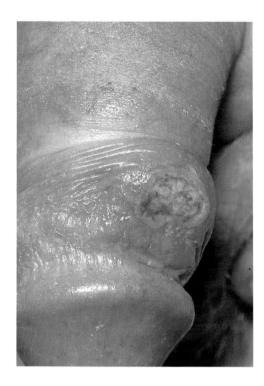

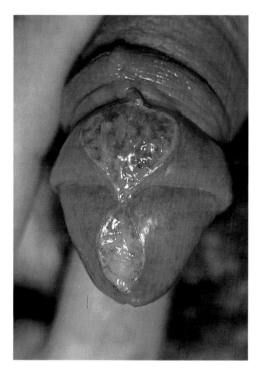

*Far left*
**10.1** Primary chancre on penis.

*Left*
**10.2** Two chancres where glans is in contact with foreskin.

## PRIMARY SYPHILIS

A single round painless ulcer (chancre) with an indurated base occurs about 3 weeks after infection (can be 10–40 days). The chancre is seen on the penis, scrotum, vulva, perianal skin or lip, but may also be found on the cervix or within the anal canal. The diagnosis should be suspected in any genital ulcer and confirmed by the demonstration of *Treponema pallidum* by dark ground microscopy. Serology (TPHA, FTA) is helpful because it becomes positive within a week of the primary sore developing.

## OTHER SINGLE GENITAL ULCERS

If the patient has been to the tropics consider **granuloma inguinale, chancroid** or **lymphogranuloma venereum**. The latter two are usually associated with marked local lymphadenopathy. All such patients should be referred to a department of genitourinary medicine where a diagnosis can be made.

Any indurated ulcer on the genitalia which is negative on dark ground microscopy should be biopsied to exclude a **squamous cell carcinoma**. An ulcer which has an odd shape or recurrent necrotic lesions should make you think of **dermatitis artefacta**.

**Genital ulcers**
**2 Multiple ulcers**

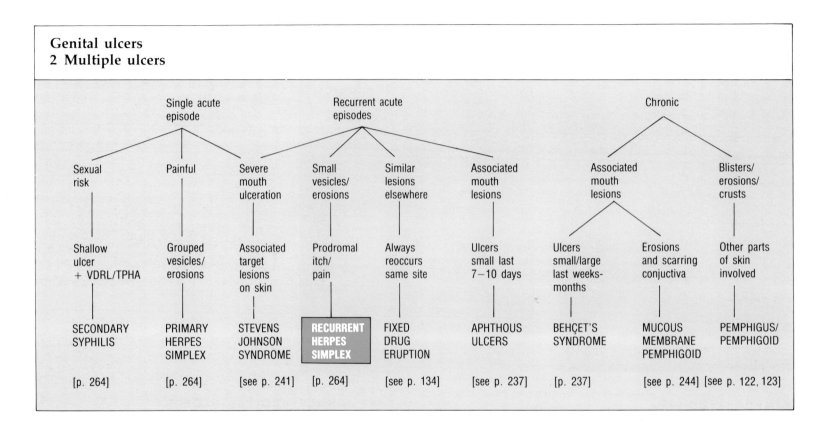

| | | | | | | | | |
|---|---|---|---|---|---|---|---|---|
| | Single acute episode | | | Recurrent acute episodes | | | Chronic | |
| Sexual risk | Painful | Severe mouth ulceration | Small vesicles/ erosions | Similar lesions elsewhere | Associated mouth lesions | Associated mouth lesions | | Blisters/ erosions/ crusts |
| Shallow ulcer + VDRL/TPHA | Grouped vesicles/ erosions | Associated target lesions on skin | Prodromal itch/ pain | Always reoccurs same site | Ulcers small last 7–10 days | Ulcers small/large last weeks– months | Erosions and scarring conjuctiva | Other parts of skin involved |
| SECONDARY SYPHILIS | PRIMARY HERPES SIMPLEX | STEVENS JOHNSON SYNDROME | RECURRENT HERPES SIMPLEX | FIXED DRUG ERUPTION | APHTHOUS ULCERS | BEHÇET'S SYNDROME | MUCOUS MEMBRANE PEMPHIGOID | PEMPHIGUS/ PEMPHIGOID |
| [p. 264] | [p. 264] | [see p. 241] | [p. 264] | [see p. 134] | [see p. 237] | [p. 237] | [see p. 244] | [see p. 122, 123] |

## SECONDARY SYPHILIS

Irregular shallow serpiginous erosions on the penis, scrotum or vulva should suggest secondary syphilis. The spirochaetes can be demonstrated in the exudate from such lesions by dark ground microscopy, and the serology will always be positive.

## HERPES SIMPLEX

This is by far the commonest cause of recurrent genital ulceration. The primary infection, usually with *Herpesvirus hominis* type 2 (but can be type 1), begins with painful grouped vesicles which rapidly break down to form erosions. The diagnosis is confirmed by finding multinucleate cell on PAP stain (see Fig. 3.10, p. 41), or by virology culture or electron microscopy if these are available.

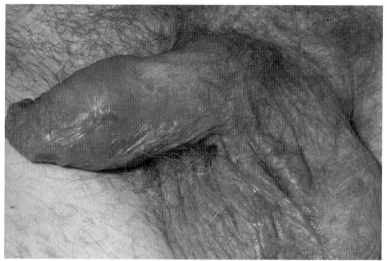

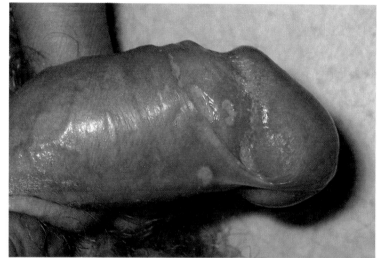

**10.3** Secondary syphilis on shaft of penis: serpiginous erosions.

Recurrent episodes of herpes simplex are common and can be precipitated by fever, stress and sexual trauma.

## APHTHOUS ULCERS

These may rarely occur on the genitalia as well as in the mouth (see p. 237).

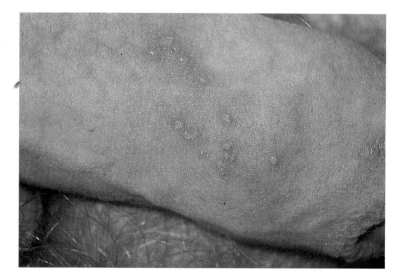

*Right above*
**10.4** Herpes simplex type 2: multiple ulcers.

*Right below*
**10.5** Herpes simplex type 2 on shaft of penis: multiple vesicles.

# Penile papules

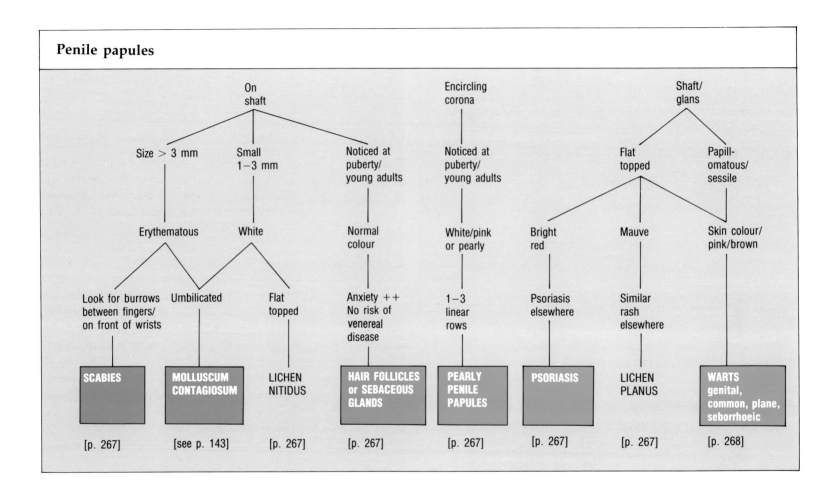

On shaft
- Size > 3 mm
  - Erythematous
    - Look for burrows between fingers/ on front of wrists → **SCABIES** [p. 267]
    - Umbilicated → **MOLLUSCUM CONTAGIOSUM** [see p. 143]
- Small 1–3 mm
  - White
    - Flat topped → LICHEN NITIDUS [p. 267]
- Noticed at puberty/ young adults
  - Normal colour
    - Anxiety ++ No risk of venereal disease → **HAIR FOLLICLES or SEBACEOUS GLANDS** [p. 267]

Encircling corona
- Noticed at puberty/ young adults
  - White/pink or pearly
    - 1–3 linear rows → **PEARLY PENILE PAPULES** [p. 267]

Shaft/ glans
- Flat topped
  - Bright red
    - Psoriasis elsewhere → **PSORIASIS** [p. 267]
  - Mauve
    - Similar rash elsewhere → LICHEN PLANUS [p. 267]
- Papill- omatous/ sessile
  - Skin colour/ pink/brown → **WARTS genital, common, plane, seborrhoeic** [p. 268]

## SCABIES

Discrete itchy red papules on the penis and scrotum are most likely to be due to scabies. There will usually be a rash on the trunk and limbs, and the diagnosis can be confirmed by finding one or more burrows along the sides of the fingers (see p. 116).

## LICHEN NITIDUS/LICHEN PLANUS

Lichen planus nearly always affects the genital area. The lesions are identical to those elsewhere: flat topped, shiny, mauve papules, polygonal in shape. If the papules are very small they are called lichen nitidus.

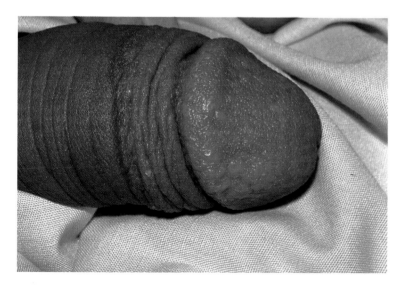

10.6 Lichen planus on glans: flat shiny mauve papules.

## HAIR FOLLICLES OR SEBACEOUS GLANDS

The normal hair follicles and sebaceous glands on the shaft of the penis may be perceived as abnormal by some adolescents and young adults. Reassurance only is required.

## PEARLY PENILE PAPULES

They are small skin coloured, pink or pearly papules 1–3 mm across, occurring around the corona in about 10% of males after puberty. Many young men go to their doctor when they first notice them thinking they are abnormal. Reassurance is all that is needed.

## PSORIASIS

The diagnosis of psoriasis on the glans or shaft of the penis is not usually difficult since the bright red colour is just like psoriasis elsewhere. On the glans the scaling will be absent, but on the shaft the plaques should have the typical silvery scaling. In boys between the ages of 5 and 15 psoriasis may first appear on the penis and cause considerable anxiety to their parents. In adults it is often a problem because of pain during intercourse and because it causes considerable anxiety and embarrassment in case their partner should think it is contagious.

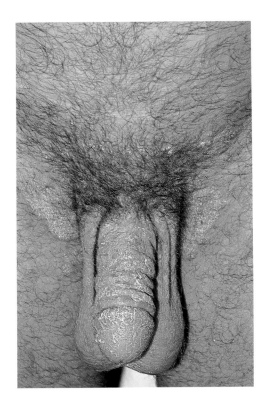

10.7 Psoriasis on penis, pubic area and groin.

sexual partner should also be checked and other sexually transmitted diseases should be looked for and excluded.

2 *Common warts*, see p. 222. ⎫ All these occur on the genitalia
3 *Plane warts*, see p. 163. ⎬ but look exactly the same as
4 *Seborrhoeic warts*, see p. 163. ⎭ similar lesions elsewhere.

5 *Condylomata lata*. Lesions that look like viral warts may occur in secondary syphilis. Individual lesions often have an eroded surface which exudes serum which is teeming with spirochaetes. Think of this if the patient is unwell and check the VDRL.

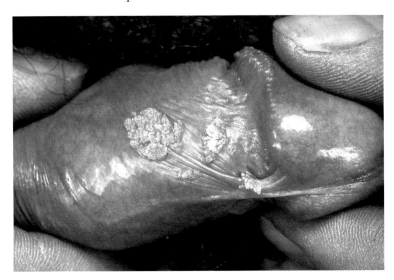

10.8 Genital warts on the shaft and prepuce; pearly penile papules around the corona.

## WARTS

Warty lesions on the penis, scrotum, vulva or perianal skin may be due to:

1 *Genital warts* (condyloma accuminata). These are due to one of the human papilloma viruses (HPV 6, 11, 16, 18) and are spread by sexual contact. These single or multiple, skin coloured, pink or brown warty papules with a moist rather than rough surface can occur anywhere on the genitalia or perianal skin. The patient's

# Papules on scrotum and pubic area

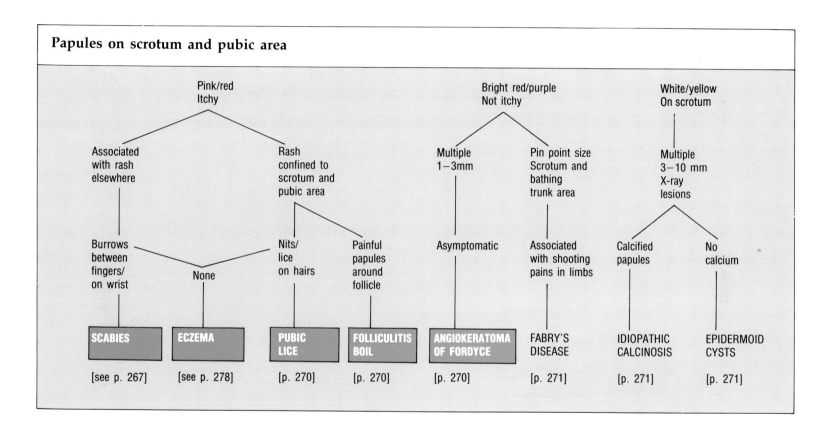

Pink/red
Itchy

Associated with rash elsewhere

Rash confined to scrotum and pubic area

Burrows between fingers/ on wrist

None

Nits/ lice on hairs

Painful papules around follicle

**SCABIES**

[see p. 267]

**ECZEMA**

[see p. 278]

**PUBIC LICE**

[p. 270]

**FOLLICULITIS BOIL**

[p. 270]

Bright red/purple
Not itchy

Multiple 1–3mm

Pin point size Scrotum and bathing trunk area

Asymptomatic

Associated with shooting pains in limbs

**ANGIOKERATOMA OF FORDYCE**

[p. 270]

FABRY'S DISEASE

[p. 271]

White/yellow
On scrotum

Multiple 3–10 mm X-ray lesions

Calcified papules

No calcium

IDIOPATHIC CALCINOSIS

[p. 271]

EPIDERMOID CYSTS

[p. 271]

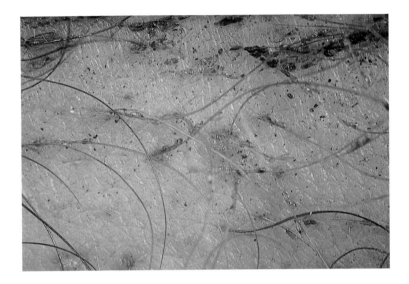

## PUBIC LICE

Itching confined to the pubic area may be due to lice. Look first for nits on the pubic hairs. These look identical to the nits which are found in the scalp; oval white shiny capsules 1–2 mm long are firmly attached to the pubic hairs. In Negroes the nits are sometimes very dark in colour but are otherwise the same. The adult louse is also firmly attached to two adjacent hairs and is quite difficult to pull off.

If no nits are present look for other signs of eczema or scabies to confirm the diagnosis of these.

## FOLLICULITIS/BOIL

Painful papules on the scrotum or pubic area are probably due to infection of hair follicles with *Staphylococcus aureus* (Figs. 4.6, 4.8, pp. 77, 80). Small red papules around hair follicles, some of which have pus in the centre are due to folliculitis. Large nodules are boils. With both there may be painful lymphadenopathy in the groin. Bacteriology culture will confirm the diagnosis.

## ANGIOKERATOMA OF FORDYCE

Angiokeratomas are dilated blood vessels with a hyperkeratotic surface. Bright red or purple non-itchy papules on the scrotum are quite common particularly in the elderly. They are usually asymptomatic, but may occasionally bleed.

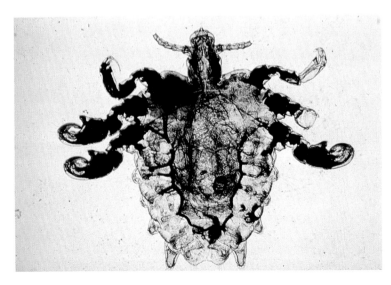

*Left above*
**10.9** Nits of pubic lice on pubic hair.

*Left below*
**10.10** Crab (pubic) louse (x 25).

## FABRY'S DISEASE (ANGIOKERATOMA CORPORIS DIFFUSUM)

This is a very rare X-linked disorder in which tiny angiokeratomas occur on the skin in the area usually covered by the underpants. They occur just before puberty and are associated with excruciating pains in the limbs and with renal failure. If this diagnosis is suspected, a specialist opinion should be sought.

## EPIDERMOID CYST AND IDIOPATHIC CALCINOSIS

Single or multiple white papules confined to the scrotal skin are most commonly due to epidermoid cysts. In women similar cysts occur on the labia majora. Histologically they are identical to epidermoid cysts elsewhere, with a lining that looks like normal epidermis and filled with keratin.

Sometimes lesions that look exactly the same as epidermoid cysts are found not to be cysts histologically but lumps of calcium lying in the dermis. There is no capsule around them and there is no indication of why they are there. They are not associated with hypercalcaemia or deposition of calcium elsewhere. If the diagnosis is thought of before excision, the calcification can be shown on X-ray. Both conditions are completely harmless.

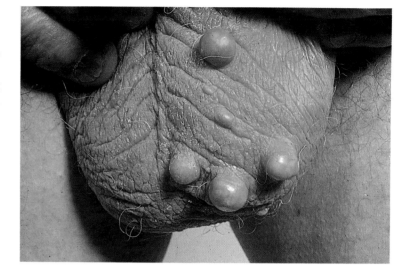

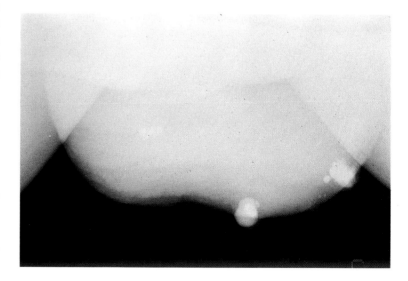

*Right above*
**10.11** Idiopathic calcinosis of scrotum. Deposits of calcium in the skin: these look identical to epidermoid cysts.

*Right below*
**10.12** Idiopathic calcinosis of scrotum: X-ray to show calcium in same patient as Fig. 10.11.

# Plaques on glans penis (uncircumcised)

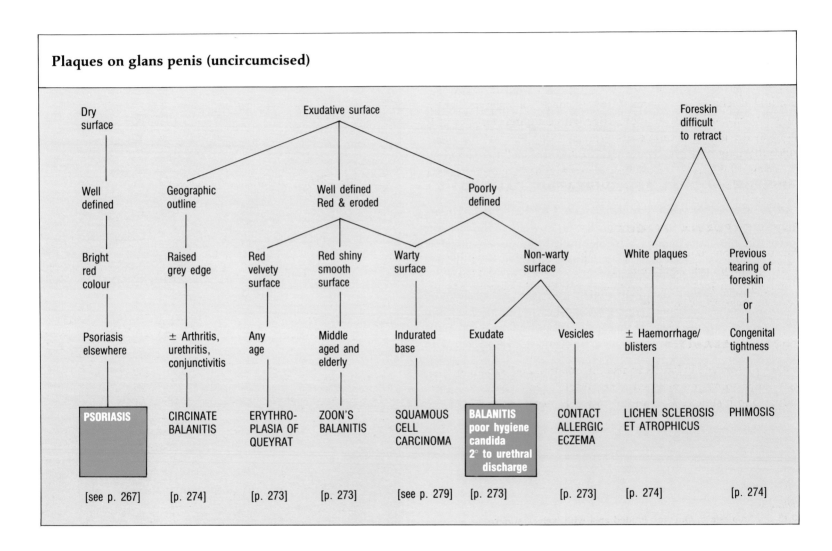

| | | | | | | | | |
|---|---|---|---|---|---|---|---|---|
| Dry surface | | Exudative surface | | | | | Foreskin difficult to retract | |
| Well defined | Geographic outline | Well defined Red & eroded | | Poorly defined | | | | |
| Bright red colour | Raised grey edge | Red velvety surface | Red shiny smooth surface | Warty surface | Non-warty surface | | White plaques | Previous tearing of foreskin or |
| Psoriasis elsewhere | ± Arthritis, urethritis, conjunctivitis | Any age | Middle aged and elderly | Indurated base | Exudate | Vesicles | ± Haemorrhage/ blisters | Congenital tightness |
| PSORIASIS | CIRCINATE BALANITIS | ERYTHRO-PLASIA OF QUEYRAT | ZOON'S BALANITIS | SQUAMOUS CELL CARCINOMA | BALANITIS poor hygiene candida 2° to urethral discharge | CONTACT ALLERGIC ECZEMA | LICHEN SCLEROSIS ET ATROPHICUS | PHIMOSIS |
| [see p. 267] | [p. 274] | [p. 273] | [p. 273] | [see p. 279] | [p. 273] | [p. 273] | [p. 274] | [p. 274] |

## BALANITIS

Balanitis means inflammation of the glans penis. It is uncommon in those who have been circumcised. It may be due to poor hygiene (particularly if the foreskin is tight and difficult to retract), urethral discharge or trauma. Always check for candida, which may not have the typical appearance with outlying pustules as it does in the groin. If candida is present, test the urine for sugar since this may be a presenting sign of diabetes mellitus in middle or old age. If it occurs very acutely consider contact allergic eczema due to condoms, spermicidal foams or applied medicaments.

## ERYTHROPLASIA OF QUEYRAT

An uncommon condition which is due to an intra-epidermal (*in situ*) squamous cell carcinoma. The surface of the red plaque in this condition looks like velvet. If in doubt a biopsy should be done to make the diagnosis.

## ZOON'S BALANITIS

Zoon's plasma cell balanitis is also uncommon, and usually occurs as a single shiny red plaque in the middle aged or elderly. Again biopsy and histology is required to reach a correct diagnosis.

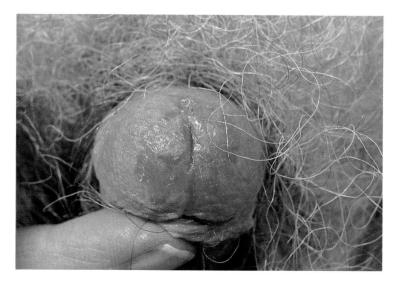

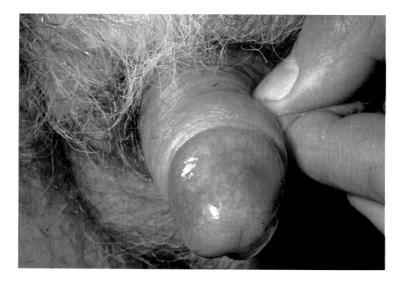

*Right above*
**10.13** Erythroplasia of Queyrat: eroded area with 'velvet' surface.

*Right below*
**10.14** Zoon's plasma cell balanitis: surface more shiny.

## CIRCINATE BALANITIS

This occurs in some patients with Reiter's disease: HLA B27 +ve arthritis, (sacro-iliitis and/or polyarthitis), urethritis or dysentery and conjunctivitis. A red eroded area occurs on the glans which spreads outwards in phases with a grey circinate edge.

## PHIMOSIS

Difficulty in retracting the foreskin in a young adult without any clinical signs may be due to a congenitally tight foreskin or repeated trauma.

## LICHEN SCLEROSUS ET ATROPHICUS

Unlike the same condition in females, lichen sclerosus et atrophicus in males most commonly affects young adults. It can present in a number of ways. The patient may notice white discolouration of the glans or prepuce, blistering or haemorrhage, difficulty in retracting the foreskin or the urine spraying out uncontrollably during micturition. On examination ivory white macules, papules or plaques are present on the glans with or without obvious atrophy. Blisters or haemorrhage may also be seen; see also p. 279.

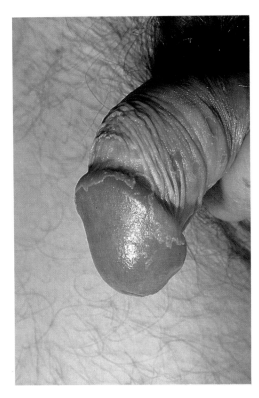

*Left*
**10.15** Circinate balanitis: eroded area with grey irregular edge in a patient with Reiter's disease.

*Right*
**10.16** Lichen sclerosus et atrophicus on glans: white atrophic areas with haemorrhagic erosions.

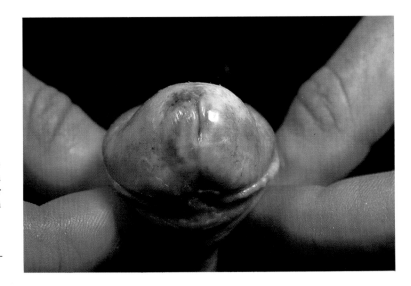

## Plaques on scrotum, shaft of penis and glans (circumcised)

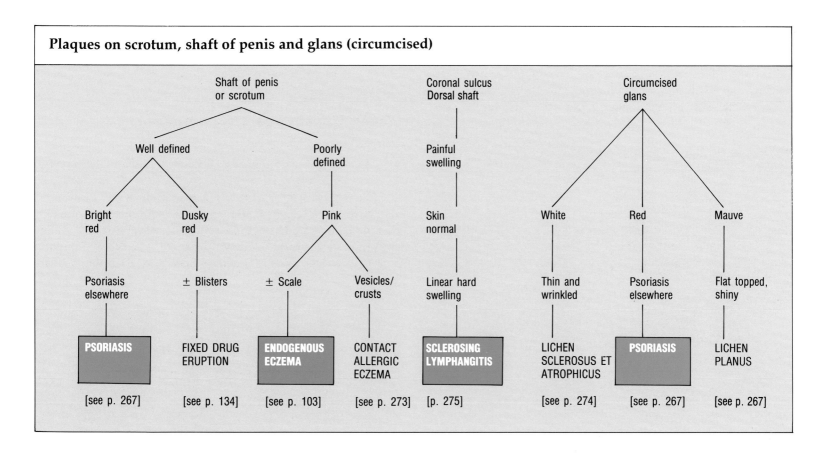

### SCLEROSING LYMPHANGITIS

A cord-like swelling following sexual intercourse around the coronal sulcus or extending down the dorsum of the shaft of the penis is not at all uncommon in young men. It is due to a lymphatic thrombosis: it is harmless and resolves spontaneously in 4–6 weeks.

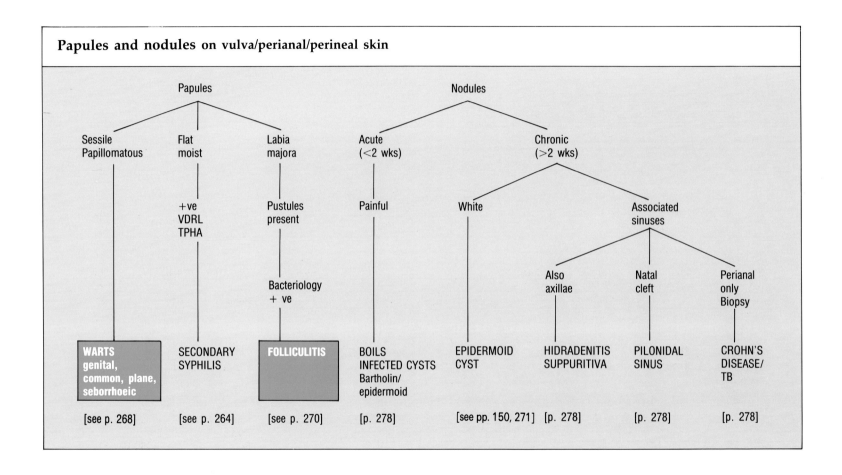

**Papules and nodules** on vulva/perianal/perineal skin

Papules

Sessile Papillomatous

Flat moist

+ve VDRL TPHA

**WARTS genital, common, plane, seborrhoeic**

[see p. 268]

SECONDARY SYPHILIS

[see p. 264]

Labia majora

Pustules present

Bacteriology + ve

**FOLLICULITIS**

[see p. 270]

Nodules

Acute (<2 wks)

Painful

BOILS INFECTED CYSTS Bartholin/ epidermoid

[p. 278]

Chronic (>2 wks)

White

EPIDERMOID CYST

[see pp. 150, 271]

Associated sinuses

Also axillae

HIDRADENITIS SUPPURITIVA

[p. 278]

Natal cleft

PILONIDAL SINUS

[p. 278]

Perianal only Biopsy

CROHN'S DISEASE/ TB

[p. 278]

## Plaques on vulva/perianal/perineal skin

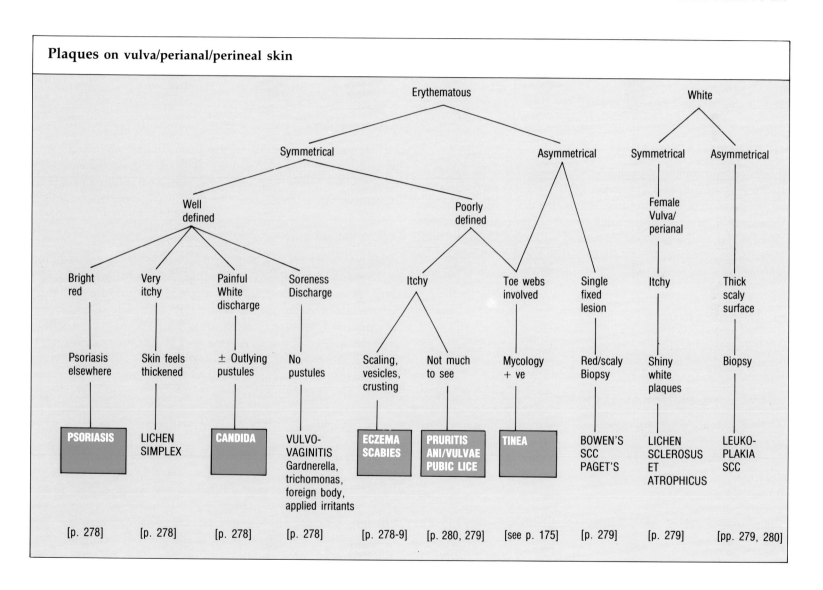

## BOILS AND INFECTED CYSTS

An acutely painful red nodule on the vulva, pubic area or scrotum may be due to an infection of a hair follicle (boil), Bartholin gland (in women) or a pre-existing epidermoid cyst.

## HIDRADENITIS SUPPURITIVA

This is an uncommon condition where painful papules, nodules, discharging sinuses and scars occur at sites where apocrine glands are present: axillae, pubic area, labia majora, scrotum, groins, perianal skin, buttocks or the areolae of the breasts. If such lesions are confined to the perianal skin think of Crohn's disease and, much less commonly, tuberculosis. A biopsy will be needed to confirm these diagnoses.

## PILONIDAL SINUS

A tender papule or nodule in the midline of the natal cleft may be due to a pilonidal sinus.

## VULVAL OR PERIANAL ITCHING

When a patient complains of perianal or vulval itching, you need to know whether there are any other symptoms such as pain or vaginal discharge, whether a rash is present on the vulva or elsewhere, and whether anyone else in the family has the same or similar symptoms.

The following rashes present with vulval itching.

### Psoriasis

This is often misdiagnosed on the vulva because it itches. If the plaque is bright red rather than pink or mauve, whether scaly or not, it is probably psoriasis. Look at the natal cleft, the rest of the skin, the scalp and the finger nails for other signs of psoriasis to confirm your diagnosis.

### Lichen simplex

Lichen simplex is a single mauve or pink thickened plaque with or without obvious excoriations. It is an area of lichenification which is due to, and kept going by, continual rubbing or scratching; see p. 98.

### Vulvo-vaginitis

Soreness rather than itching is usually the presenting symptom of *candidiasis* of the vulva. An acute vulvitis with a red glazed appearance (Fig. 6.6, p. 177) is characteristic and there may be an associated thick white vaginal discharge. The diagnosis can be confirmed by direct microscopy (Fig. 1.3, p. 10), or culture of the discharge. If positive, remember to test the urine for sugar. If negative, think of an anaerobic infection with Gardnerella, trichomonas infection or a retained foreign body in the vagina as possible causes.

### Eczema

*Atopic eczema* or unclassifiable *endogenous eczema* may present with vulval itching. In the former, intolerable genital itching may be the final straw that makes it impossible for the patient to cope with her eczema. In the latter, sexual infidelity or anxiety about possible venereal disease may be the precipitating factor. Both conditions are clinically identical to eczema elsewhere with poorly defined, itchy, pink papules and plaques with excoriations and scaling but no vesicles; see p. 103.

*Contact irritant eczema* occurs in babies in the form of nappy rash: an identical rash can occur in the elderly if they are incontinent. Applied irritants may produce an irritant eczema or an acute vulvitis.

*Contact allergic eczema* is most often due to deodorants, contraceptives or medicaments containing lanolin, parabens (preservative), antibiotics or local anaesthetics. It usually presents acutely with vesicles, weeping and crusting, and it may be extremely sore rather than itchy. Patch testing will be needed once the acute reaction has settled down to sort out the cause.

### Scabies

There should be an itchy rash all over the body except on the face, and the tell-tale burrows will be found between the fingers. Other members of the family or sexual contacts may also be itching. See p. 116.

### Pubic lice

The diagnosis is confirmed by finding nits on the pubic or labial hair. See p. 270.

### Tumours

A single red scaly plaque unresponsive to treatment should be biopsied to exlude Bowen's disease, extramammary Paget's disease or a squamous cell carcinoma (SCC).

### Lichen sclerosus et atrophicus

This is a very itchy condition which principally occurs on the vulva and perianal skin. It occurs in little girls or in middle-aged women. In children itching, soreness or blisters are the presenting symptoms; it gets better spontaneously at puberty. In older women intolerable itching, soreness or dyspareunia are the reasons for seeking help. White atrophic papules and plaques with or without follicular plugging or haemorrhagic blisters are seen on the vulva or perianal skin. Occasionally lesions may occur elsewhere on the skin where they are very similar to lichen planus with flat-topped, polygonal papules with a wrinkled atrophic surface, but white in colour rather than mauve.

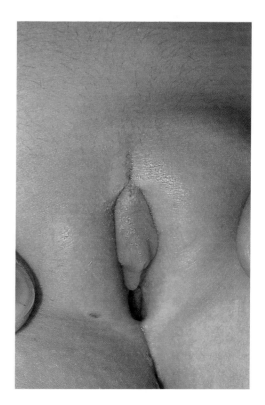

10.17 Lichen sclerosus et atrophicus on vulva of young girl.

White plaques on the vulva which are thickened rather than atrophic may be due to **leukoplakia** (see p. 246). If in doubt a biopsy will distinguish between leukoplakia and lichen sclerosus.

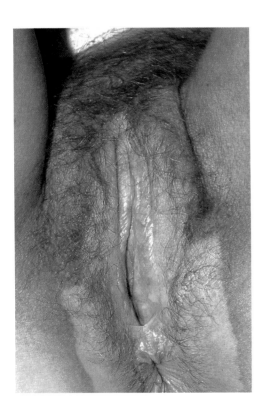

**10.18** Lichen sclerosus et atrophicus on vulva of middle aged lady.

**Pruritis vulvae**

When no rash is present consider:

1 The rash has temporarily got better: see the patient again when it reoccurs.

2 *Threadworms*. These usually cause pruritis ani in children, but in females may wander forward to the vulva causing itching there too. The diagnosis is made by seeing the worms wriggling out of the faeces (tell the patient or mother to look), by seeing them on the perineum, or by the Sellotape test (apply some sticky transparent tape to the perianal skin, place on a glass slide and look for the threadworm ova).

3 *Psychological*. In adults the cause of vulval itching when there is nothing to see may be due to a psychosexual problem, particularly if symptoms follow intercourse.

**Pruritis ani**

The causes of pruritis ani are very similar to those of pruritis vulvae, but it occurs in both men and women. In addition discharge from the anus can cause itching due to the area being continually wet. Mucous discharge, bleeding or diarrhoea can all cause problems and a rectal examination is essential to exclude a carcinoma of the rectum.

# Chapter 11
# Nails

## ANATOMY OF THE NAIL

Nails are keratin produced by a modified epidermis called the nail matrix. From this grows the nail plate (Fig. 11.1), which lies on the nail bed. Nails protect the end of the digits and on the fingers are useful for picking up small objects and for scratching. Abnormalities can arise from any part of the nail apparatus.

**Nail apparatus**

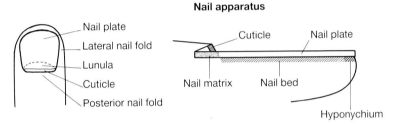

**11.1** Anatomy of the nail.

## EXAMINATION OF THE NAIL

### Procedure

When looking at the nails examine the following in turn:

### End on

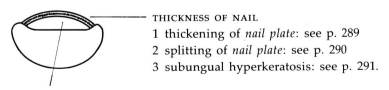

THICKNESS OF NAIL
1 thickening of *nail plate*: see p. 289
2 splitting of *nail plate*: see p. 290
3 subungual hyperkeratosis: see p. 291.

DETACHMENT OF NAIL FROM NAILBED (*onycholysis*) Abnormality of hyponychium: see p. 290

### From above

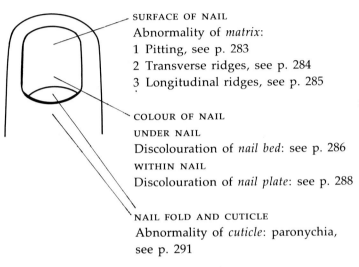

SURFACE OF NAIL
Abnormality of *matrix*:
1 Pitting, see p. 283
2 Transverse ridges, see p. 284
3 Longitudinal ridges, see p. 285

COLOUR OF NAIL
UNDER NAIL
Discolouration of *nail bed*: see p. 286
WITHIN NAIL
Discolouration of *nail plate*: see p. 288

NAIL FOLD AND CUTICLE
Abnormality of *cuticle*: paronychia, see p. 291

### From side

SHAPE OF NAILS
1 Over curvature, see p. 292
2 Spoon shaped nails, see p. 292
3 Wedge shaped nails, see p. 292
4 Ingrowing toenails, see p. 293

LOSS OF NAILS
1 Without scarring (temporary), see p. 293
2 With scarring (permanent), see p. 293

LUMPS AND BUMPS AROUND NAILS
See p. 293

## ABNORMALITIES OF NAIL MATRIX

### Pitting

Inflammatory conditions affecting the matrix cause areas of abnormal keratin to be formed, which become detached from the nail plate leaving pits or ridges. Pits are more easily seen in finger nails than in toe nails.

*Causes*
1  Isolated pits may be found in normal nails.
2  Psoriasis: small regular pits (see Fig. 11.2).
3  Eczema: larger and more irregular pits (see Fig. 11.4); associated with eczema around the nail.
4  Alopecia areata: small regular pits (may be a poor prognostic sign for regrowth of hair).

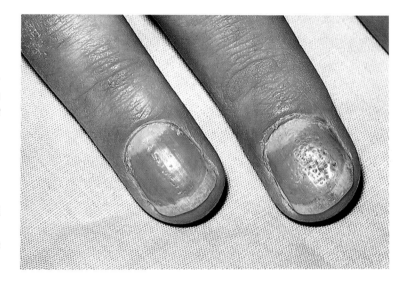

**11.2** Pitting of the nails in psoriasis.

**11.3** Pathology of psoriasis and eczema in the nails.

(a) Pathology of psoriasis
When these changes occur in the nail matrix there will be well defined areas of parakeratosis in the nail plate, which fall off easily after minor trauma leaving well defined pits.

(b) Pathology of eczema
When these changes occur in the nail matrix, because the areas are less well circumscribed, the pitting is larger and more irregular, so that there may be longitudinal or transverse ridges rather than pits.

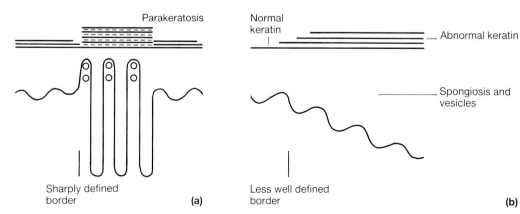

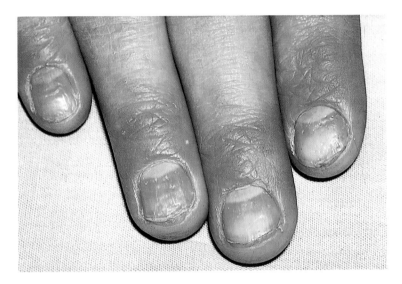

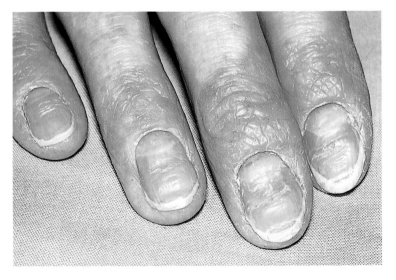

## Transverse ridging

*Causes*

1  Eczema: some pits are so broad as to form transverse ridges.
2  Chronic paronychia: due to pressure on the nail matrix.
3  Beau's lines: a single line at the same place in all the nails is due to cessation of growth of the nail matrix at the time of a severe illness. When this is over, the matrix will begin to function

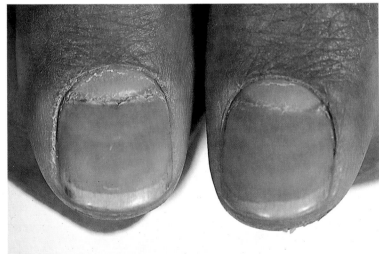

**11.6** Beau's lines.

*Left above*
**11.4** Pitting of the nails in eczema.

*Left below*
**11.5** Pitting and transverse ridges in eczema: note the eczema on the fingers around the nails.

normally and the nail will grow out with a line in it. Finger nails grow at a rate of approximately 1 mm/week (toenails at about half that speed), so you can tell how long ago the illness was.

## Longitudinal ridging

*Causes when all nails affected*
1   A few ridges are seen in normal nails.
2   Lichen planus: fine regular lines.
3   Darier's disease: regular fine lines with notching of the end of the nail.

*Causes when a single nail affected*
1   Median nail dystrophy: looks like an upside down Christmas tree. It is a temporary abnormality and gets better spontaneously after a few months. The cause is unknown.
2   Habit tic deformity: differs from median nail dystrophy in being a broader groove made up of numerous concave transverse ridges. It is due to picking or biting the nail.
3   A single wide groove may be due to a myxoid cyst or wart over the posterior nail fold which is pressing on the underlying matrix (see Fig. 11.11).

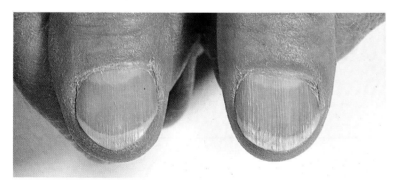

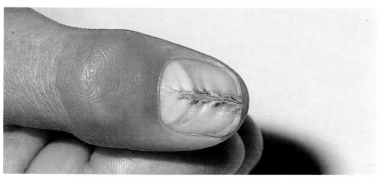

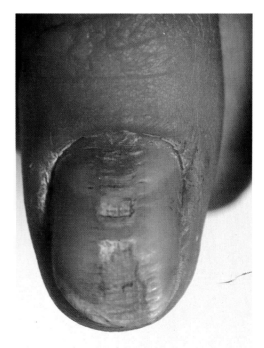

*Left above*
**11.7** Longitudinal ridging due to lichen planus.

*Left below*
**11.8** Median nail dystrophy.

*Right*
**11.9** Habit tic deformity.

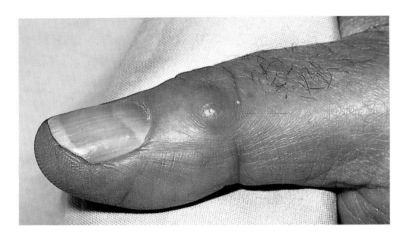

*Above*
**11.10** Myxoid (mucous) cyst.

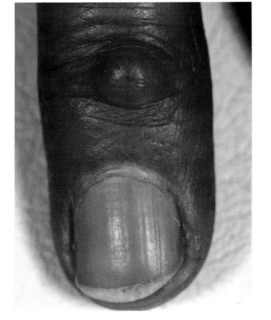

*Left*
**11.11** Longitudinal groove in nail due to myxoid cyst pressing on the nail matrix.

## ABNORMALITIES OF NAIL BED

### Discolouration under the nail

The nail bed is the epidermis underneath the nail. In normal circumstances it does not produce keratin. Problems in the nail bed cause areas of discolouration under the nail.

*Causes*

### Orangy-brown colour (called *salmon patches*)
Due to psoriasis.

### Red/purple/black colour
1 Splinter haemorrhages are small red longitudinal streaks. They are classicaly seen in subacute bacterial endocartitis, but are, in fact, so common as to be unreliable clincial sign.

**11.12** Salmon patch and onycholysis in a patient with psoriasis.

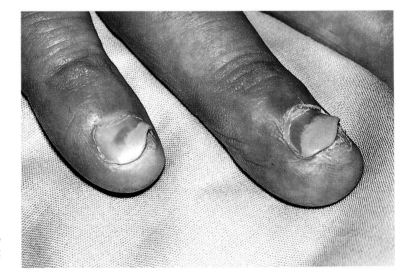

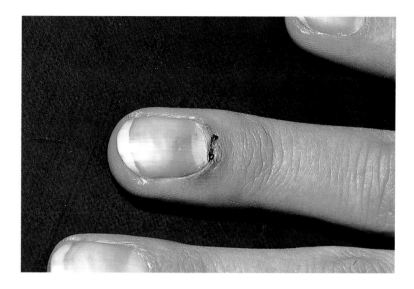

2 Subungual haematoma results from bleeding under the nail following trauma. It can occur on finger or toe nails. Initially the area is exquisitely painful and dark red/purple in colour. With time, if the blood is not released immediately by puncturing the nail, the area is discoloured black or brown. It can be distinguished from a subungual malignant melanoma by making a small horizontal nick on the nail plate at the distal end of the discolouration and watching for a week: a subungual haematoma will grow out at the same rate as the nail so the nick will still be at the distal end of the discolouration; a melanoma does not grow at such a regular rate.

## Brown colour

A round or oval brown area is a junctional naevus of the nail bed. If it is growing or made up of different colours consider a malignant melanoma.

## Pink/mauve colour

A glomus tumour is a rare benign tumour that presents as a tender area under the nail, particularly on pressure or in the cold.

## White colour

Pallor of the nail bed occurs in hypoalbuminaemia or chronic renal failure.

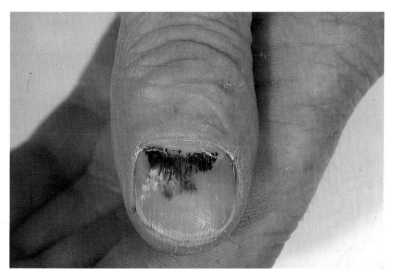

*Left above*
**11.13** Acute subungual haematoma.

*Left below*
**11.14** Subungual haematoma: this appearance could be confused with a subungual malignant melanoma (see Fig 11.17 and 11.31).

## ABNORMALITIES OF NAIL PLATE

No nail thickening—if nail thick see tinea, p. 289

### Discolouration of the nail plate

*Causes*

1 External staining especially from nicotine and medicaments, less commonly from hair dyes or tints in nail varnish.

2 Drugs: chloroquine stains the nails blue-grey, penicillamine stains them yellow; all nails should be equally affected.

3 White nails:

(a) small white streaks due to minor trauma occur in most people at some time.

(b) familial leuconychia where the whole of the nail is white; inherited as an autosomal dominant trait.

(c) distal end of nail white and lifted off = onycholysis, see p. 290.

4 Brown lines in nail. If the line is a thin one down the entire length of the nail it will be due to a junctional naevus of the nail matrix. A broad line under the nail which is expanding in width or extending up through the nail should make you think of a malignant melanoma.

5 White/yellow. An irregular discoloured area associated with a thickened nail plate is likely to be due to tinea.

6 Yellow nail syndrome. All the nails are yellow or green in colour. They are excessively curved in both longitudinal and trans-

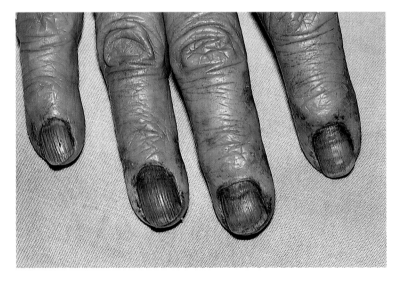

**11.15** Brown staining of nails from potassium permanganate.

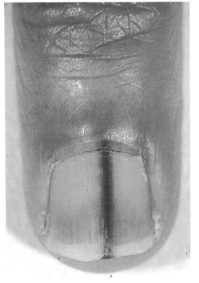

**11.16** Junctional naevus of nail matrix.

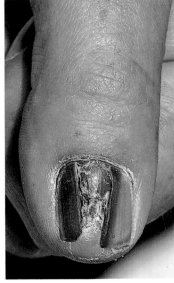

**11.17** Malignant melanoma of nail bed.

verse directions, and the rate of growth is slowed almost to a standstill: sometimes onycholysis occurs too. It is thought to be due to a congenital abnormality of the lymphatics, although the nail changes do not occur until adult life and often not until middle or old age. There may be other abnormalities of the lymphatics such as lymphoedema of the legs or bilateral pleural effusions.

### Thickening of nail plate itself

*Causes*

1 Tinea. Dermatophyte fungi live on keratin and so multiply within the nail plate, causing it to become thickened, and discoloured white or yellow. They can only become established in

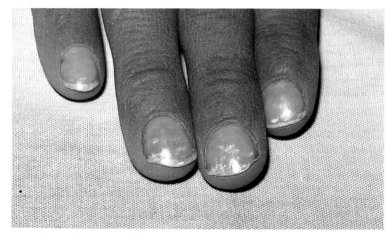

11.18 Normal white streaks in nails.

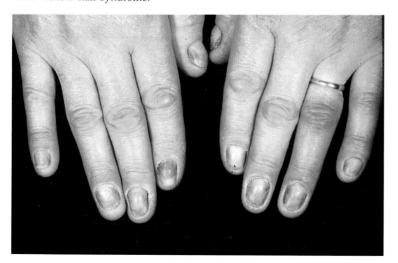

11.19 Yellow nail syndrome.

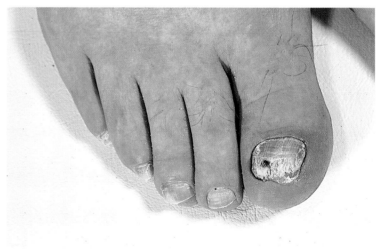

11.20 Tinea of right great toe nail: note the thickening of the nail plate and no onycholysis.

nails that are growing slowly, so affect toenails much more readily than fingers nails. Once established the rate of growth slows down even more so that cutting the affected nails becomes an infrequent necessity.

It can be difficult on the feet to distinguish clinically between thickening of the nails due to tinea, and onycholysis and subungual hyperkeratosis due to psoriasis. First look at the finger nails: the changes of psoriasis will be more obvious there, with associated pits, salmon patches and onycholysis. If the finger nails are not involved, tinea is more likely: on the toes not all the nails are affected, the disease is asymmetrical and you can look between the toes or on the instep for other evidence of fungal infection. Nail clippings for direct microscopy or fungal culture can also be done.

2 Chronic trauma, particularly to toenails, can produce thickened nails.

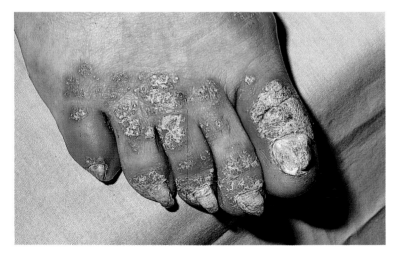

**11.21** Psoriasis of toe nails: subungual hyperkeratosis.

### Splitting of the ends of the nails

1 Lamellar splitting occurs when the distal portion of the nail plate splits into horizontal layers. It is mainly seen in women and is due to damage to the keratin from water and detergents.
2 Longitudinal splitting may occur along a longitudinal ridge.

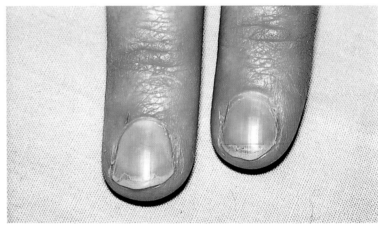

**11.22** Lamellar splitting at distal end of nail plates.

## ABNORMALITIES OF THE HYPONYCHIUM

### Onycholysis

This means separation of the nail plate from the nail bed. It is due to an abnormality of the hyponychium where the nail plate is less firmly stuck down onto the nail bed.

*Causes*

1 Trauma. On the hands the commonest cause is over manicuring. Damage occurs to the hyponychium by cleaning underneath the

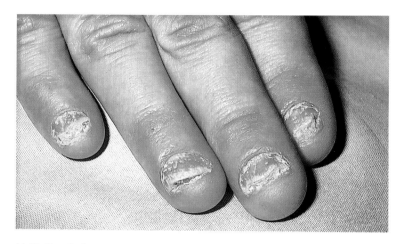

**11.23** Onycholysis and subungual hyperkeratosis in a patient with psoriasis.

nails with a nail file. On the feet it usually follows a subungual haematoma.

2   Psoriasis, seen more obviously on finger nails than toe nails. Once the nail has lifted off, *subungual hyperkeratosis* occurs and it may be difficult to distinguish this from thickening of the nail plate due to tinea (see p. 289 and compare Figs. 11.20, 11.21 and 11.23).

3   Poor peripheral circulation.

4   Thyrotoxicosis.

5   Contact allergic eczema to substances which penetrate through the nail plate, e.g. PTBP formaldehyde resin used as glue for sticking on artificial nails.

## ABNORMALITIES OF THE CUTICLE

The cuticle is an area of keratin joining the skin of the posterior nail fold to the nail plate preventing bacteria and yeasts from getting into the tissues around the nail. If the cuticle is lost (usually due to chronic trauma to hands that are continually wet, or to eczema), infection can occur under the posterior or lateral nail folds to cause paronychia. There are two types:

### Acute paronychia

This is due to infection with *Staphylococcus aureus* (less commonly *Streptococcus pyogenes*). There is exquisite pain, a bright red swelling and pus formation.

Rarely *herpes simplex* may be the cause, but grouped vesicles over the distal phalanx are the giveaway sign.

### Chronic paronychia

*Candida albicans* produces a more chronic infection with less swelling, a duller red colour, and no pus. The nail plate may show

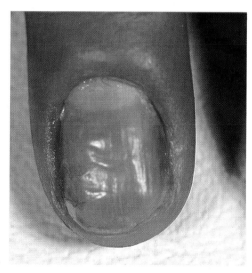

**11.24** Chronic paronychia.

transverse or longitudinal ridges from chronic pressure on the nail matrix. Secondary invasion with bacteria such as *Pseudomonas aeroginosa* may cause green discolouration of the nail. If the hands are kept away from water for several months, cuticle regrowth will occur.

## ABNORMALLY SHAPED NAILS

### Over curvature

1   Clubbing is an apparent overcurvature of the nail due to loss of the angle between the posterior nail fold and the nail plate. If there is any doubt, put the distal phalanges of the two thumbs together: there should be a diamond-shaped gap between them. This disappears if the nails are clubbed. If clubbing is present look for chronic chest disease, carcinoma of the bronchus or congenital heart disease.
2   Overcurvature due to resorption of the distal phalanx in hyperparathyroidism; the nail curves over the end of the finger.
3   Yellow nail syndrome, see p. 288.

### Spoon shaped nails (koilonychia)

Most often seen in association with iron deficiency anaemia (although most patients with iron deficiency do not have this change). It may be a normal finding in young children.

### Wedge shaped nails

Pachyonychia congenita is a rare genetic abnormality in which the nail grows both vertically and horizontally causing a thick wedge shaped nail, which is unsightly on the fingers and causes pain from pressure of shoes on the feet.

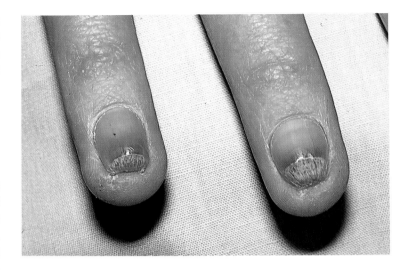

11.25 Pachyonychia congenita: wedge shaped nails.

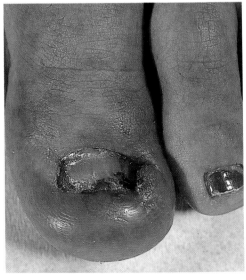

11.26 Ingrowing toe nail.

### Ingrowing toenails

Penetration of the lateral nail fold by the nail itself or a spicule of the nail causes redness, tenderness, pus formation and later granulation tissue. The great toe nail is most commonly involved. It is due to wearing shoes that are too tight and cutting the nails in a half-circle instead of straight across. Similar changes occur as a side effect of the retinoid drugs.

## LOSS OF NAILS

### Without scarring (temporary)

1   Trauma, especially to the great toe nails. Finger nails too can

be lost after a large subungual haematoma.
2   Beau's lines, after a severe illness the nail may break off at the line (see p. 284).

### With scarring (permanent)

1   Lichen planus. The cuticle grows down over and through the nail plate resulting in permanent scarring: this change is called pterygium.
2   Genetic abnormalities: all rare.

## LUMPS & BUMPS AROUND THE NAIL

1   Viral warts. Small skin-coloured, grey or brown papules with a

**11.27** Pterygium in a patient with lichen planus: this causes permanent scarring.

**11.28** Viral warts around nails.

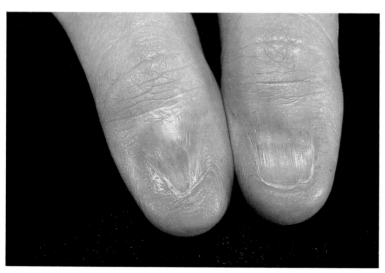

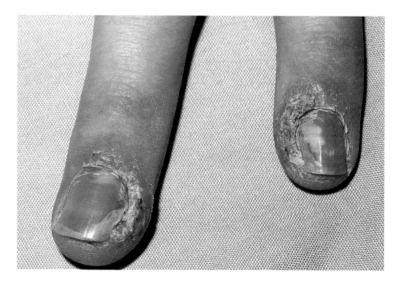

rough warty surface may occur on the skin around the nail.

2 Myxoid cyst. A round skin coloured papule over the dorsal surface of the distal phalanx (see Figs. 11.10 & 11.11, p. 286). If pricked it discharges a sticky clear fluid.

If viral warts or myxoid cysts occur over the nail matrix, they can cause a longitudinal groove in the nail plate.

3 Subungual and periungual fibromas. Small, firm, pink papules protruding from the posterior nail fold or from under the nail occur in patients with tuberose sclerosis. They appear first after puberty.

4 Subungual exostosis. This is a localized outgrowth of bone which presents as a subungual skin-coloured papule. If in doubt X-ray the digit.

5 Tumours. Rarely a squamous cell carcinoma or a malignant melanoma occur around the nail. Any inflammatory condition around a single nail which does not improve with treatment is an indication for biopsy.

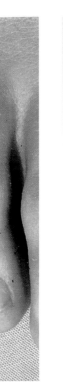

**11.29** Periungual fibroma in a patient with tuberose sclerosis.

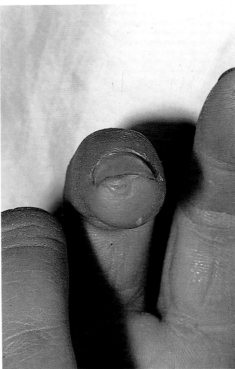

**11.30** Subungual exostosis.

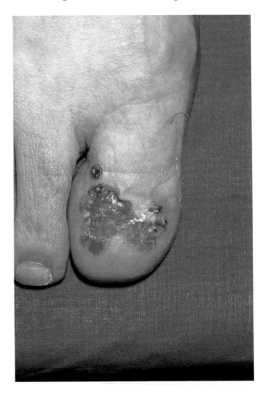

**11.31** Malignant melanoma arising in the nail bed.

# General Index

# Index of algorithms

| Surface changes | Type of lesion | Colour | Face/ bald scalp | Trunk/ arm/ thigh | Dorsum hand/ forearm | Lower leg/ calves | Axilla/ groin/ natal cleft | Dorsum foot | Palm | Sole |
|---|---|---|---|---|---|---|---|---|---|---|
| | | | | | | | | Site | | |

**Non-erythematous lesions** (usually chronic)

| Surface changes | Type of lesion | Colour | Face/ bald scalp | Trunk/ arm/ thigh | Dorsum hand/ forearm | Lower leg/ calves | Axilla/ groin/ natal cleft | Dorsum foot | Palm | Sole |
|---|---|---|---|---|---|---|---|---|---|---|
| Smooth/ normal | Macules and patches | Brown/blue/grey | | | | | | | | |
| | | present since birth | 126 | 126 | 126 | 126 | 181 | 126 | 126 | 126 |
| | | appeared after birth | | | | | | | | |
| | | all lesions <3cm size | 129 | 129 | 218 | 129 | 129/181 | 129 | 129 | 231 |
| | | some lesions >3cm size | 133 | 133 | 133 | 201 | 133 | 201 | – | – |
| | | White | 136 | 136 | 136 | 136 | 136 | 136 | 136 | 136 |
| | | Pink/red – see erythematous | | | | | | | | |
| | | Purpuric | – | 202 | 202 | 202 | – | 202 | – | – |
| Smooth/ normal | Papules (<5mm size) | Skin colour/pink/yellow | 140 | 140 | 140 | 140 | 140 | 140/219 | – | – |
| | | White/cream | 142 | 142 | 142 | 142 | 142 | 142 | 219 | 219 |
| | | Brown | 151 | 151 | 218 | 151 | 181 | 151 | 218 | 231 |
| | | Blue/black/grey/purple/ red/orange | 156 | 156 | 156 | 156 | 156 | 156 | 231 | 231 |
| | | Purpuric | – | 202 | 202 | 202 | – | 202 | – | – |
| | Papules (>5mm size)/ plaques/ nodules | Skin colour/pink/yellow/white/cream | | | | | | | | |
| | | situated on surface | 145 | 145 | 145 | 145 | 179 | 145 | – | – |
| | | situated under surface | 149 | 149 | 149 | 149 | 179 | 145 | 219 | 219 |
| | | Brown | 151 | 151 | 218 | 151 | 181 | 151 | 218 | 231 |
| | | Blue/black/grey/purple/red/orange | | | | | | | | |
| | | no recent size increase | 156 | 156 | 156 | 156 | 156 | 156 | – | 231 |
| | | recent size increase | 158 | 158 | 158 | 158 | 158 | 158 | – | – |
| | | Purpuric | – | 202 | 202 | 202 | – | 202 | – | – |
| Warty | –″– | Skin colour/brown | 161 | 161 | 218/221 | 161 | 161 | 161 | 221 | 231 |
| Scaly/ horny/ rough | –″– | Skin colour/brown | | | | | | | | |
| | | single/few (1–5) lesions | 167 | 167 | 221 | 167 | 167 | 167 | 211/221 | 231 |
| | | multiple/widespread lesions | 164 | 164 | 164 | 164 | 164 | 164 | 211 | 224/225 |
| Crust/ exudate/ bleeding | –″– | Any colour | | | | | | | | |
| | | single/few (1–5) lesions | 171 | 171 | 171 | 171 | 171 | 171 | 171 | 171 |
| | | multiple/widespread – see chronic erythematous | | | | | | | | |
| Ulcerated | –″– | Any colour | 171 | 171 | 171 | 193/197 | 171 | 193/197 | 171 | 193/197 |
| Macerated | –″– | Any colour | – | – | – | – | – | – | – | 224/225/231 |
| Hairy | | Brown | 172 | 172 | 172 | 172 | 172 | 172 | – | – |

| Surface changes | Type of lesion | Number of lesions | Face/ bald scalp | Trunk/ arm/ thigh | Dorsum hand/ forearm | Lower leg/ calves | Axilla/ groin/ natal cleft | Dorsum foot | Palm | Sole |
|---|---|---|---|---|---|---|---|---|---|---|
| | | | | | | | | | | |

**Acute erythematous lesions/rash**

| Surface changes | Type of lesion | Number of lesions | Face/ bald scalp | Trunk/ arm/ thigh | Dorsum hand/ forearm | Lower leg/ calves | Axilla/ groin/ natal cleft | Dorsum foot | Palm | Sole |
|---|---|---|---|---|---|---|---|---|---|---|
| Smooth/ normal | Transient lesions/swelling (last < 24 hours at one site) | | 35 | 72 | 72 | 72 | | | | |
| | Widespread progressive maculo-papular rash | | 74 | 74 | 74 | 74 | | | | |
| | Fixed lesions/rash – NO PUSTULES | single/few lesions | 77 | 77 | 206 | 186 | 179 | 223 | 211 | 224 |
| | | multiple/widespread | 35 | 78 | 207 | 186 | 174/179 | 223/186 | 211 | 224 |
| | | generalized rash (> 50% body surface involved) | 82 | 82 | – | – | – | – | – | – |
| | PUSTULES present | | 79 | 79 | 79 | 79 | 179 | 79 | 211 | 224 |

Scaling—see chronic erythematous lesions/rash

| Surface changes | Type of lesion | Number of lesions | Face/ bald scalp | Trunk/ arm/ thigh | Dorsum hand/ forearm | Lower leg/ calves | Axilla/ groin/ natal cleft | Dorsum foot | Palm | Sole |
|---|---|---|---|---|---|---|---|---|---|---|
| Blisters/exudate crusts/erosions | Localized | | 39 | 39 | 39 | 39 | 39 | 39 | 211 | 224 |
| | Widespread | | 44 | 81 | 81 | 81/186 | 174 | 81/186 | 211 | 224 |
| | Generalized | | 82/122 | 82/122 | – | – | – | – | – | – |